Daily Vagus Nerve Exercises:

A Self-Help Guide to Stimulate Vagal Tone, Relieve Anxiety and Prevent Inflammation with Practical Exercises to Release your Body's Natural Ability yo Heal

Sherman Sander

© **Sherman Sander Copyright 2019 - All rights reserved.**

The contents of this book may not be reproduced, duplicated or transmitted without direct written permission from the author.

Under no circumstances will any legal responsibility or blame be held against the publisher for any reparation, damages, or monetary loss due to the information herein, either directly or indirectly.

Legal Notice:

This book is copyright protected. This is only for personal use. You cannot amend, distribute, sell, use, quote or paraphrase any part or the content within this book without the consent of the author.

Disclaimer Notice:

Please note the information contained within this document is for educational and entertainment purposes only. Every attempt has been made to provide accurate, up to date and reliable complete information. No warranties of any kind are expressed or implied. Readers acknowledge that the author is not engaging in the rendering of legal, financial, medical or professional advice. The content of this book has been derived from various sources. Please consult a licensed professional before attempting any techniques outlined in this book.

By reading this document, the reader agrees that under no circumstances is the author responsible for any losses, direct or indirect, which are incurred as a result of the use of information contained within this document, including, but not limited to, — errors, omissions, or inaccuracies.

Table of Contents

Introduction *6*

Chapter 1 What is Vagus Nerve *11*

Chapter 2 Main Functions of the Vagus Nerve *18*

Chapter 3 How the Vagus Nerve Affects Anxiety *24*

Chapter 4 How the Vagus Nerve Affects Stress *31*

Chapter 5 Vagus Nerve and Inflammation *36*

Chapter 6 Vagus Nerve and Depression *39*

Chapter 7 Signs Your Vagus Nerve Requires Attention *46*

Chapter 8 Activating the Vagus Nerve and Exercises *52*

Chapter 9 Passive Method to Activate the Vagus Nerve *60*

Chapter 10 Creating a Vagal Tone Routine *64*

Chapter 11 Meditative Techniques for the Support of the Vagus Nerve 70

Chapter 12 Measuring Nervous Function with Heart Rate Variability (HRV) *76*

Chapter 13 (VNS) Vagus Nerve Stimulation *79*

Chapter 14 Practical Exercises to Stimulate the Vagus Nerve *85*

Chapter 15 Health And Life Benefits of Vagus Nerve Stimulation *91*

Chapter 16 Vagus Nerve Stimulation to Heal from PTSD *97*

Chapter 17 Vagus Nerve Stimulation to Heal from Trauma *102*

Conclusion *107*

Introduction

Nervousness can be tricky. It's outlandishly muddled, profoundly close to home, and ridiculously difficult to foresee. There are times when we think our uneasiness is behind us—that we are at last one stage ahead—yet something happens, and we are on our heels once more, battling to return to a position of harmony and quiet. We are on the understudies of our uneasiness, and that is the reason seeing precisely how our sensory system functions—and what we can do to quiet it—can be staggeringly enabling.

In any case, what does "quieting your sensory system" indeed mean? Numerous individuals would depict it as easing back the pulse, developing the breath, and loosening up various muscles. But what associates these sensations to the mind? Enabling us to acquaint you with the vagus nerve, the piece of the body that appears to clarify how our psyches control our bodies, how our bodies impact our brains, may give us the instruments we have to quiet them both.

Post-traumatic stress disorder (PTSD) is brought on by people who have experienced a traumatic injury or languish trouble or functional disability. Manifestations incorporate sentiments of re-encountering the horrendous mishap, keeping away from tokens of the damage, uplifted tension and excitement, and negative musings or emotions. Ongoing catastrophic events, mass shootings, psychological oppressor assaults, and urban communities under attack add to the worldwide weight of PTSD which, as indicated by a recent report, influences 4–6% of the world's population, even though most of the injuries identified with mishaps and sexual or physical savagery. Shockingly, there is no known fix, and flow medicines are not convincing for all patients. A PTSD psychopharmacology committee recently gathered and distributed their accord proclamation, calling for a quick activity to address the emergency in PTSD treatment, referring to three significant concerns.

The US FDA endorses just two medications (sertraline and paroxetine) for the treatment of PTSD. These meds decrease side effects seriousness; however, it may not create a total reduction of side effects. The subsequent concern is identified with polypharmacy. PTSD patients are recommended prescriptions to address every one of their numerous extraordinary and assorted side effects, including nervousness, trouble dozing, sexual brokenness, wretchedness, and interminable torment. The high comorbidity among PTSD and fixation gives further difficulties to pharmacotherapies. The third significant concern is the absence of headways in the treatment of PTSD; no new prescriptions have been endorsed since 2001.

Going past side effect alleviation, the 'best quality level' way to deal with treating PTSD pathology is introduction based treatment, where patients are presented to the tokens of the injury until they figure out how to connect these prompts with wellbeing. Despite the fact that there is proof for adequacy with this methodology, not all patients react entirely to the treatment. Introduction treatment relies on the way toward stifling the adapted dread memory, which is overwhelmed by another mind that creates through rehashed exposures. The patients with nervousness issues and PTSD show weaknesses in their capacity to quench adapted feelings of dread, which could add to the advancement of scatters and may meddle with the progress in treatment. Since the memory of the injury isn't lost at the same time, but rather, upgrades through treatment based on newly learned affiliations that horrible rival alliances, the parity of the two recollections can move after some time, prompting backslide. Different difficulties incorporate the trouble in perceiving and smothering apprehension of every single molded boost and a high dropout rate, which isn't astonishing given that shirking is one of the indications of PTSD.

Numerous creature investigative labs have tried endeavors to create adjunctive medications to quicken or improve the impacts of presentation-

the wake of preparing. In this way, VNS alone isn't adequate to decrease the dread reaction. These discoveries recommend that VNS may diminish nervousness, however, matching explicit pliancy and memory tweak is vital for elimination upgrade. Our ongoing, unpublished findings show that rodents are bound to investigate the open arms of a rodent raised in addition to labyrinth following getting VNS, proposing that VNS produces a powerful anxiolytic impact. Moreover, corticosterone levels expanded radically in trick treated rodents following testing on the raised in addition to the labyrinth, however, such an expansion was not seen in VNS-treated rodents. This work ought to be imitated in different settings, yet it is an empowering initial move toward distinguishing an assistant treatment that may improve decency and adequacy in presentation-based treatments.

Chapter 1

What is Vagus Nerve

We know that the Vagus nerve is a long, "wandering" nerve; it is a parcel of sensory and motor fibers. It begins in the brain stem and interacts with the heart, lungs, and gut. It continues to spread out and interact with other major organs such as the liver, gallbladder, spleen, and more.

Our involuntary nerve center is boosted and regulates insensate body operations. It monitors your heart rate, breathing, food digestion, and sweating. Our blood pressure and blood glucose are balanced. It helps the function of the kidney, the discharge of testosterone and bile, the release of saliva is stimulated, controls taste releases tears, and is a major key in orgasms in women and fertility issues (Ropp, 2017).

Approximately 80 percent of the nerve fibers transmit information by way of four "lanes" of the nerve. In the opposite direction, the fifth lane is simultaneously bringing signs from the brain through the body.

The nerve begins in the brain stem, extends down the neck and into the chest where it splits into left and right Vagus. Tens of thousands of nerve fibers that each "road" is composed of branches out into all the major organs in the body.

To say that the Vagus nerve has a lot to do with how our involuntary nerve center is powered is an understatement. It has been noted that "if we were without the Vagus nerve, many major functions of the body that keep us alive would not be maintained." In order to have your Vagus functioning at optimum levels, it needs to be activated.

Acetylcholine, the neurotransmitter stimulates muscle contractions and is used by the Vagus nerve. This allows signals to be moved from one place to another and stimulates various organs. Acetylcholine production can be interfered with by substances such as Botox and the heavy metal mercury.

Botox is a substance that can interfere with the Vagus nerve. Another problem is mercury - it blocks acetylcholine.

What happens if your Vagus nerve is not functioning properly? For some of us, the solution may be to have it electronically stimulated.

The FDA has approved the use of vagus nerve stimulation in treating two different chronic conditions. People who have epilepsy or have an autistic child may find that this route is the most beneficial way to stimulate the Vagus nerve to treat and improve these illnesses. Scientists have recognized the possibility of stimulating the Vagus nerve with an electronic implant that is activated with a magnetic strip. Chronic conditions such as epilepsy and autism have had FDA approval to implant this device for treatment. Those with chronic conditions report great results having their Vagus nerve stimulated many times each day.

People with chronic pain and stiffness and who could barely get out of bed are seeing amazing results. They're able to go on long walks, swim, and even dance again. The stimulation of the Vagus nerve is aiding the body in doing what it's supposed to do – heal itself.

When our nervous system functions at optimum levels, we feel great. However, Vagus nerve damage or low vagal tone is more the norm. Even small changes to the Vagus nerve can exhibit results that are impressive. There are several studies being conducted to prove the stimulation of the nerve is a useful way to treat more chronic diseases. Whether the treatment is electronic or non-invasive, stimulations proving to be a non-medicinal way to have diseases show improvement. However, what about stimulating the Vagus nerve ourselves? What can we do to activate it? But before we get into how to activate it, a look at what causes the nerve to become damaged is called. Fixing what's broken doesn't work if you don't address and fix what caused it to be broken in the first place.

Vagal Dysfunction

Vagal dysfunction can bring a myriad of problems that can disrupt the normal flow of the body and introduce chronic disease and illness.

The Vagus nerve has quite a few conditions that have been linked or are being researched at this time for a link to this nerve. These issues can range from minor conditions to serious, more significant issues.

Quite a few people will have a vasovagal reaction eventually because of the overstimulation or stress of the Vagus nerve.

Some reasons and results linked to the Vagus nerve being irritated or damaged include:

- Obesity
- Hormonal imbalance
- Constant stress and anxiety
- Alcohol addiction
- Diabetes
- Cancer
- Spicy foods
- IBS (Irritable Bowel Syndrome)
- Insomnia
- Chronic Fatigue
- Chronic inflammation
- Depression
- Tinnitus
- Migraine headaches
- Alzheimer's disease
- Poor blood circulation
- Leaky gut
- Mood disorders

- Vitamin deficiency

So, if you're overweight, are stressed and anxious on a consistent basis, overdo it with alcohol, have developed diabetes, eat spicy foods, are constantly fatigued, and can identify with many of the other causes or reactions you may be having, your Vagus nerve is probably irritated. These conditions are due to the inability to switch from the sympathetic responses and reestablish balance and calmness in your body.

Damage of the Vagus Nerve

A range of symptoms can manifest due to damage to the Vagus nerve. The main reason for this is because the nerve is so long and affects many organs of the body. (Seladi-Schulman, 2018)

- A hoarse voice or wheezy
- Loss of gag reflex
- Trouble drinking liquids
- Difficulty speaking
- Decreased production of stomach acid
- Vomiting or nausea
- Pain or abdominal bloating
- Testing the Vagus Nerve

A doctor may check the gag reflex to test the Vagus nerve. The doctor may use a cotton swab to tickle both sides of the back of the throat. Normally, this should cause a person to gag. If they don't, this may indicate a problem with the Vagus nerve.

There are ways that can help to revitalize the Vagus nerve. Stimulation of the nerve can be a help for your body. Studies have been done to exhibit how important the Vagus nerve is and how it interfaces with so many of the body's organs.

The Vagus nerve furnishes us to react to psychological, physical, and emotional symptoms that come from a lack of balance in the body and might be the key to improving your health.

When you perform vagal nerve stimulation, there are major improvements health-wise, including the relief of many autoimmune illnesses and an overall feel-better effect.

The Vagus nerve works well when it is strong and has a high vagal tone. If you are dealing with many of the named irritants and results linked to the vagal nerve, the vagal tone is low.

Vagal tone is an indication of the condition you are in. For example, people who exercise on a regular basis, athletes, and those who practice yoga or other types of physical activity will exhibit a higher vagal tone. Adversely, people who are alcoholics or drink far beyond legal limits, along with people who are bedridden or don't exercise regularly, have lower vagal tone. You may have a low vagal tone if your mother also had a low vagal tone during her pregnancy with you. She may have been stressed, anxious, or angry during the pregnancy. It's possible the low vagal tone was passed down to you.

In order to increase your vagal tone, you need to work it out, just like exercising the body and continue to activate it. You don't need to do an elaborately long workout – 15 to 20 minutes each day would be good. The more you do, it would be better, but if you're doing daily stimulations of the Vagus nerve, you're doing okay.

Activating the Vagus Nerve

Most people envision the Vagus nerve to be one thin cord reaching from the brain stem to the gut. Actually, it is a nerve that extends down both sides of the body and is a branch of the shaggy, meandering nerve that connects to most of the major organs like a system of cables or roots. (Zimmerman, 2019)

The Vagus nerve is responsible for the mind-body connection, its role as a go-between between thinking and feeling.

Stimulating the Vagus nerve has an impactful effect on lowering the heart rate. This is what relaxes us. Our Vagus nerve is receiving information from the way we breathe and sends it to the brain and the heart the message our breathing signifies.

The more we activate it with deep breathing, the more we negate the effects of the sympathetic nervous system. Instead of feeling stressed and anxious, we feel calm and relaxed.

The heart slows, and we relax when we breathe slowly, but when we breathe quickly, our heart rate increases, and we feel anxious or amped. Vagal activity is at its highest, and the heart rate is at its lowest when you exhale.

Researchers found that the most calming way to breathe is six times a minute. Five seconds inhale, five seconds exhale.

This style of slow breathing is also what practitioners of meditation naturally drift into with mantras they recite slowly. Each time you repeat a meditation mantra, your breathing naturally coordinates your breathing at six times a minute. (Zimmerman, 2019)

There are ways to measure the vagal tone – finding out how strong, healthy, and functioning the nerve is. Measuring the heart rate variability (HRV) is a substitute way to measure vagal tone (the other way would be open chest surgery).

The amount that the heart rate fluctuates between breaths in when it speeds up naturally and breathe out when it slows down is heart rate variability. Thus the heart rate increases when we inhale and decreases when we exhale, and the difference between the two rates measure vagal tone.

People who are physically active such as athletes, usually have a higher vagal tone, and those who have a sedentary lifestyle with little to no exercise and, surprisingly, astronauts who spend time in no-gravity situations are known to have low vagal tone.

There are many ways to stimulate the Vagus nerve. You can laugh, sing, chant, hum, gargle, meditate, do full-body exercising, breathing exercises,

or engage in sound-related activities such as listening to music or white noise. These are just a few activities recommended for stimulation. Splashing cold water on your face or taking a full-body rinse with cold water after a shower is another way of stimulating the Vagus nerve.
Mild exercise and general full-body exercise will increase fluids in the gut, which will stimulate the Vagus nerve. The muscles at the back of the throat will be worked by laughing and singing, also activating the nerve and sounding OM while practicing meditation.
Activating the Vagus nerve encompasses sound. Sound is a major alternative in healing, as well as music. They are a great way to stimulate the Vagus nerve in a non-invasive, natural manner.
Dancing is another physical activity that releases endorphins, reduces stress, and causes our body to have a feeling of optimism, happiness, and calm. It also incorporates two key elements – sound and movement, which are good for Vagus stimulation.
Dance, as movement therapy, reduces anxiety, helps people suffering from depression, and those who have anxiety in social settings. It increases strength in muscles and improves flexibility offering a better range of motion.
It also increases core strength, thus improving coordination, balance, and posture.
Aside from being a good overall exercise, it stimulates the brain helping to reduce feelings of loneliness, memory (remembering dance steps) recognizing beat, synchronizing music with movement, and feeling the rhythm of the music.

Chapter 2
Main Functions of the Vagus Nerve

We would like to underscore further the importance of taking proper care of the nervous system, thereby ensuring the proper functioning of the vagus nerve and associated biological systems.

The vagus nerve is one broad highway that conducts the flow of information from the biological systems that it controls up to the CNS. It is the primary raison d'etre of the vagus nerve. The vagus nerve is like a central command post in which the information comes and goes. Consequently, the vagus nerve provides the CNS with all of the data; it needs to keep the body alive.

Let's assume that the vagus nerve simply stops working for whatever reason. In such a situation, the person would simply die. How so? If the vagus nerve ends sending information to the CNS, the CNS may conclude that the heart and lungs have stopped functioning. Therefore, the brain may have no choice but to begin shutting down other organ systems as well. This type of response may lead doctors to place a patient on life support.

This example highlights the importance that the vagus nerve has on the body's overall ability to sustain life. Now, let's assume that the vagus nerve is functioning correctly, but there is some kind of damage to one of the organ systems. In that case, the vagus nerve relays the data on the damage to the organ system back up to the CNS. The brain then sends back the information through the vagus nerve and adjusts accordingly. For instance, if one lung is severely damaged, the brain may choose to shut down that lung and shift all of the breathing functions to the other healthy lung. This is enough to keep the body alive though not necessarily at peak performance.

In addition, the vagus nerve is the central command post for the digestive system. This is a crucial function to consider since the digestive system provides the body with the nutrition it needs to repair itself, fuel movement, and keep cells running along. Hence, the digestive system needs close attention. This causal link between the digestive system and the CNS explains why folks who have undergone a traumatic experience and experience gastrointestinal distress. When the nervous system suffers a significant jolt, it is not uncommon to see that it has severe repercussions for the entire network controlled by the vagus nerve.

So, let's move on and take a more in-depth look at the specific functions that are associated with the vagus nerve.

The Visceral Somatic Function

Given the fact that the vagus nerve is part of the Autonomic Nervous System (ANS), it is linked to the entire body. Think of it as the main highway that receives traffic from all over the region even if the majority of motorists don't actually plan to stay in that particular area. In a way, the primary transportation is just passing through.

Based on that premise, any disruption in the flow of traffic in that area may lead to confusion in the flow of traffic in other seemingly unrelated areas. The same goes for the nervous system and biological functions.

When we refer to a bodily function, we are talking about the reaction that comes as a result of the stimuli in the environment surrounding an organism. In this case, the human body is the organism immersed in a given situation.

As such, the physical function that the vagus nerve plays is one of constant monitoring and regulation. Think of it as one large pressure valve that looks to regulate the build-up within a large engine. If too much pressure builds up, then the driver may explode. The same goes for the nervous system.

With that in mind, there is one interesting bit of good news. The body is adept at adjusting to its environment. So, if the individual finds themselves consistently inundated by stressful situations, there is the possibility that the body will become acclimated to such levels of stress. In a way, it creates a "new normal."

An example of this attitude can be seen in the so-called "adrenaline junkies." These people become addicted to extreme sports due to the exhilaration that they get from engaging in a dangerous activity. However, they consistently need to up the ante since their nervous system continually adjusts to the level of danger in each event. So, in order to get the same rush, they need to overload their nervous system more and more. Otherwise, they may not find the same amount of enjoyment in the same activities.

As far as the physical function is concerned, the vagus nerve is continuously tracking the performance of the body's internal organ systems. As a matter of fact, it is designed with a number of automatic switches that are intended to protect the body from grievous damage. Think of these switches like circuit breakers in an electrical system. When the system is overloaded by the electrical current, the circuit breaker is tripped, thereby protecting the entire system. If no such switch existed, the wiring would overheat potentially causing a fire.

The vagus nerve has built-in parameters that prevent the body from overexerting itself to the point where permanent damage is done to organs. Consider this situation:

A person who has been working non-stop for a week may find that after going on little to no sleep, they simply crash and sleep for an extended period of time. This reaction is triggered in the nervous system in order to prevent the heart from literally burning out. This is why drug consumption, the kind that disrupts the nervous system, making it prone for individuals to suffer from cardiac arrest. Since the substance wreaks havoc with the PNS natural regulation mechanisms, the body keeps going until it eventually shuts down.

An excellent example of this can be seen in modern cars. The car's computer shuts the engine down when it diagnoses a potentially dangerous problem in the engine. The car's control computer module shuts off the flow of gas, for example, in order to keep the engine from completely failing. The vehicle will restart once the issue has been corrected.

So, just like a car's control module, the vagus nerve serves as the body's central regulation unit. This protects the body's vital organs from failing altogether, at which point death would ensue. This is why optimal performance from the vagus nerve is essential to ensuring the body's overall optimal performance.

The Physical Motor Function

Since the vagus nerve is part of the overall ANS, it is also connected to the body's peripheral nervous system, which controls the movement of limbs. As such, the vagus nerve is involved in the motor functions of the body.

Now, the vagus nerve itself does not regulate movement, but it does control the biological functions that aid movement. The following example will illustrate this point.

When a person engages in physical activity, the CNS broadcasts the necessary signals to the limbs for movement, be it running, swimming, and so on. However, the heart is also responsible for supply blood to the muscles while the lungs need to provide oxygen. Furthermore, there is an increased metabolic response as the body needs to create the energy it requires to sustain the level of physical activity. If the action exceeds the heart's capacity to pump blood and the lungs' ability to provide oxygen, then the individual may simply get tired and stop moving.

This example highlights how vital the vagus nerve is when taking the movement into account. High-performance athletes have trained not only for their sport, but also develop stamina. Now, you may have heard of this term, yet it is generally associated with endurance, that is, sustaining physical activity over more extended periods of time. But the fact of the matter is that stamina is the body's ability to provide the elements the body needs to sustain prolonged periods of physical activity.

Consequently, the vagus nerve is able to recognize these increased levels of physical activity and make the necessary adjustments so that muscles get the elements they need in order to keep going. It should be noted that the vagus nerve will also recognize when an athlete is becoming overexerted. At which point, the athlete may feel like they can't go on anymore. This is the body's protective measures that keep it from causing severe damage.

This last point illustrates the importance of keeping a balanced nervous system so that the vagus nerve can perform its functions appropriately, thereby allowing the body's organ systems to provide the elements that the body requires.

Essential Biological Functions

These functions are what basically keeps the body alive. After all, if your heart stops breathing, then chances are you are not going to make it.

With that in mind, it is essential to note that when the vagus nerve is not functioning at 100%, that is, when there is some kind of disruption, the crucial biological systems may begin to go haywire. In some cases, it might be a slow and progressive disruption, while in other cases, it may be a sudden and shocking disruption.

Let's consider two possible scenarios:

An individual who has been working a stressful job begins to feel the effects of chronic stress over months or even years of accumulated stress. Suddenly, they may develop cardiac conditions, anxiety, or even chronic digestive disorders. Yet, the progression of these conditions was so subtle that the person didn't really feel much of a difference.

On the flip side, there is a person who underwent a major traumatic incident; for instance, the loss of a loved one. The stress caused by the sudden loss of a dear person may cause a sudden overload to the nervous system. This sudden overload may lead to the onset of any of the aforementioned conditions. This may prompt swift intervention by medical professionals in order to address the beginning of the symptoms the person is experiencing.

In either case, the vagus nerve can come under attack. At this point, there is a severe need for treatment that can correct the imbalances in the nervous system, thus promoting recovery from the overwhelming effects on the nervous system. In fact, you may be surprised that some of the most common conditions that you may be familiar with can be addressed by balancing out the vagus nerve's functions.

Chapter 3
How the Vagus Nerve Affects Anxiety

Anxiety is something that every person will experience in life, and it is entirely reasonable. We feel anxiety when we go to a job interview or on our first date. However, when you suffer from an anxiety disorder, things can be very different.

It might start with a sense of dread, and you may begin to feel fearful or irritable, you can't make it go away no matter what you do. An anxiety disorder is different from merely feeling anxious every now and then. Those that suffer from an anxiety disorder struggle with day to day tasks such as going to work or checking out at the grocery store. They may not be able to socialize or be part of a relationship.

Types of Anxiety

As stated, there are many different types of anxiety; however, there are only six major types of anxiety disorder. They are PTSD or post-traumatic stress disorder, generalized anxiety disorder, social anxiety disorder, OCD or obsessive-compulsive disorder, panic disorder, and finally, phobia.

PTSD, as most people know post-traumatic stress disorder, occurs as a result of someone having a life-threatening or traumatizing event take place in their life. The person could experience agitation, nightmares, random flashbacks or recollections, paranoia, and evasion of any circumstance that would remind them of the event.

OCD or obsessive-compulsive disorder is something that we hear thrown around a lot, but many people really do not understand. OCD is much more than just wanting to clean your house every day or make sure that the pictures are straight. It is compulsions that the patient has no control over, such as turning the light on and off 36 times before they are physically able to leave the room, and if the light is turned off 35 times, they have to start over.

Generalized anxiety disorder is also known as GAD, happens when a patient worries so much or has so many fears that they are unable to accomplish tasks for the day to day life. They may also feel that something terrible is always going to happen no matter what. When someone is a worrywart, they are demonstrating symptoms of GAD. They have no reason to feel anxious, they have no history of bad things happening to them, but the fear is so intense that they are not able to focus on anything else.

Social anxiety disorder is when a person has an extreme fear of negativity when they are in public or a fear of being humiliated in public. Someone who is excessively bashful may be suffering from a social anxiety disorder; however, it may become even more extreme than that. Sometimes the person will also withdraw from their families. They are so afraid that they do not want to interact with people at all. Those who have stage fright are often used as an example of what social anxiety looks like.

We have all heard of phobias, a fear that is exaggerated concerning something that would or could not pose any type of danger or threat to the person. A hatred is very intense, and people will go to extremes to ensure that they avoid the thing that they are afraid of. In reality, this is only reinforcing the fear; however, many people have phobias of heights, specific animals, flying, or of the dark.

All of the different types of anxiety disorders can be placed in one of these major types. While they are all anxiety disorders, it is crucial to know the difference because they all affect the person differently and can affect different areas of their lives.

Symptoms of Anxiety

Anxiety not only affects a person's mental health, but it can impact them physically as well. While we know that there are short term effects of anxiety, what many people do not know is that there are short term effects as well.

- Symptoms of anxiety can include:
- Feeling fearful, nervous, or even tense
- Feeling restless
- Suffering from panic attacks
- Increased heart rate
- Increased breathing rate
- Shaking
- Sweating
- Weakness or fatigue
- Dizziness
- Trouble concentrating
- Insomnia
- Digestive issues and nausea
- Problems with body temperature (such as feeling far colder or hotter than is usual)
- Pains in the chest
- Feeling the need to display certain behaviors in order to reduce the anxiety that is felt

Moreover, anxiety affects the body in many other ways, which can actually lead to chronic illnesses.

When our bodies feel stress, they respond by telling our bodies that we are going to have to flee or fight. This is known as the fight or flight response.

At this point, our bodies also release both adrenalin and cortisol, which many people know as the stress hormones.

While the fight or flight response is constructive if you are hiking through the woods and come upon a bear, it is not that useful when it happens during a job interview or on a date. It is also unhealthy for us to remain in this state for an extended period of time. When we are exposed to cortisol and adrenaline for too long, they can actually cause damage to our bodies.

When we are faced with anxiety in a stressful situation, it is normal for our breathing to become faster and shallow. It allows our body to take in more oxygen so that it is prepared if we have to fight or run. If this happens all of the time, as it does when a person is suffering from an anxiety disorder, they may continuously feel lightheaded, weak, faint, or dizzy.

Anxiety can also cause our heart rates to increase as well as increase the amount of blood that is pumped through our bodies. This happens as our body is preparing to fight or run because the extra blood is going to provide our muscles with extra nutrients and oxygen. At this point, our blood vessels will also narrow, which causes hot flashes.

Our bodies begin to sweat in order to cool down, and if a person is suffering from anxiety, they may feel freezing all of the time.

After looking at what anxiety does to the cardiovascular system, it is easy to understand how an anxiety disorder could cause heart problems. Studies have actually shown that those who suffer from anxiety disorders are actually at a higher risk of developing heart disease in life.

Anxiety will boost your immune system in the short term; however, it is possible for it to have the opposite effect on the body when exposure is prolonged.

Cortisol will stop the body from releasing histamine into the body when it goes into the fight or flight reaction, and this impairs the body's immune system responses. However, it has been found that people who suffer from chronic anxiety disorders are more likely to catch the flu, a cold, or other viruses. Therefore, it is imperative that if you are suffering from any type of chronic anxiety disorder, you focus on boosting your immune system as much as possible.

When our bodies go into the fight or flight response, processes that are nonessential for survival stop, this means that digestion stops. On top of that, because adrenaline reduces blood flow to the stomach and causes it to relax, digestion is affected. Because of this, people who suffer from chronic anxiety disorders may suffer from the feeling of a churning stomach, nausea, diarrhea, or they may simply lose their appetite.

Some studies have linked anxiety, depression, and stress to IBS (irritable bowel syndrome).

Anxiety can also cause a person to feel as if they need to urinate more often. This is very common when a person has a phobia. It is believed that the body loses control of the bladder functions when the person suffers from anxiety because it is easier for the body to run from the threat if the bladder is empty. However, many scientists are still unsure why the urge to urinate happens; yet, they have many different theories.

Suffering from anxiety can have many adverse short-term effects, but it can also have long-term effects as well. Those that suffer from chronic anxiety may also have insomnia, digestive issues, depression, and difficulty in socializing, at work, or at school, substance abuse, thoughts of suicide, and a loss of interest in sex or other things that they once enjoyed. These long-term effects can be life-altering and very difficult for a person do deal with. Being a female. It is more likely for a female to suffer from anxiety than a male.

- A history of substance abuse.
- Having to deal with a lot of stress for an extended period of time, from home, finance, and/or work
- Having a parent that suffers from anxiety.
- Suffering a traumatic experience in your life.
- Having a chronic medical condition such as cardiovascular disease.
- Use of certain medications.
- Having one or more other mental health disorders.

In order to be diagnosed with an anxiety disorder, you have to see a doctor. They are the only ones that can tell you what is really going on. They will be able to provide you with the medication, support, and information about lifestyle changes you can make to feel better.

You can then focus on stimulating the vagus nerve to improve even more.

Anxiety and the Vagus Nerve

When the vagus nerve is stimulated, it causes a response, which reduces stress. Vagus nerve stimulation helps to reduce the heart rate as well as blood pressure. It also stimulates functioning in different parts of the brain as well as digestion, which allows us to feel more relaxed. This is all known as the vagal response.

Simply put, the vagal response is what happens when the vagus nerve is stimulated. When the nerve is stimulated, it helps to reduce anxiety. Amazingly yoga masters were using these techniques long before scientists even knew about the vagal response.

Researchers have found that by stimulating the vagus nerve regularly anxiety, as well as stress, can be reduced. On top of this, it can also help reduce the symptoms or even neutralize COPD, asthma, and heart disease.

This should provide us with some comfort, at least. These researchers are quickly learning that not only is our physical health entirely in our control, but our mental health is as well. Studies have shown that people who suffer from mental disorders, as well as chronic illnesses such as COPD, actually benefit from vagus nerve stimulation.

There is actual science to back up the vagal response. We talked just about the fight or flight response and how it can put a person on edge. This is the same response that you feel when a person cuts you off while you are driving or when the cashier can't seem to ring up your order right no matter how many times she tries.

This response has helped to keep the human race alive over the years, but as we learned, it can also cause a lot of damage when it is experienced too often. It is then when we do not feel that we are ever really able to relax that we need to start stimulating the vagus nerve.

While stimulating the vagus nerve may sound like it is going to be very complicated, the truth is that it really is not that hard. The good news is that it also gets easier the more that you do it. We are going to talk about how you can stimulate your vagus nerve, but let me give you a little bit of a heads up. If you can breathe, you can.

Chapter 4
How the Vagus Nerve Affects Stress

Body Stress and Vagus Nerve

Stress is a natural way of reaction to change that the body has to go through. A person is stressed when they face conflicting thoughts or when they feel threatened. If you are in a situation where you think that your life is in danger, you are likely to experience stress. Stress is accompanied by varied physical, emotional, and mental responses. When you are afraid of something or worried about something, the body will prompt specific actions to take place naturally.

Although stress is a normal part of life, it brings varied ups and downs. It is not possible to take care of your nerves if you are always afraid. As a matter of fact, any time stress kicks in, and you should let the nervous system take full control. You may experience pressure from your thoughts, your body, or the environment. In either case, the vagus nerve will directly be affected.

As we have already mentioned above, any activity that leads to either direct or indirect stimulation of the vagus nerve may affect its health. If you are always stressed, the chances are that you may continuously keep on hurting your vagus nerve. We have seen that chronic inflammation only occurs after a long time of natural rehabilitation. If the body keeps on trying to rehabilitate worn-out tissues due to injuries, it will eventually lead to inflammation. The same case applies to stress. If you continuously experience stress, you are likely to stimulate the vagus nerve to such an extent that it is impossible to recover. But how exactly does body stress relate to the vagus nerve?

Any time you are under stress, you suffer from anxiety or panic attacks. Although the symptoms of either anxiety or panic attacks are not visible, it is clear that people who suffer stress may experience some form of anxiety. The brain is programmed to respond to such stressful situations by producing CRF hormones. Although the brain naturally produces such hormones, stressful situations lead to increased production of the hormones. The CRFs travel through the hypothalamus to the pituitary glands, where they cause the release of another hormone, known as ACTH. This hormone consequently travels through the bloodstream to the adrenal glands. This leads to the stimulation of cortisol and adrenal reaction, which helps protect the boy from stress. As you can see, this process of stress protection is long and directly affects your vagus nerve. When we are suffering from stress, we are likely to get deep into a state of depression if the vagus nerve and the brain get overwhelmed.

Stress and depression have all been linked with inflammatory brain response. In other words, the process of responding to stress puts the brain under extreme pressure, leading to injuries and inflammation. In other cases, the same applies to the vagus nerve. As the nerve is exposed to the stress of trying to deal with the anxious situation, it is common for the nerve to experience injuries.

Such injuries attract the natural healing process of the body, which eventually results in inflammation. Even though the body naturally fights injuries, continued stress can lead to the constant production of hormones, which ultimately leads to actions that may cause stress to the vagus nerve.

Chronic stress can also lead to an increase in the production of glutamate in the brain. The output of glutamate may directly affect the brain and, as a result, affect the vagus nerve. For instance, glutamate is a neurotransmitter that causes migraines and depression when produced in excess. When you are under stress, it is common for the brain to initiate the production of this neurotransmitter. To protect yourself from such conditions and to ensure that you preserve your vagus nerve from any damage, ensure that you reduce stressful moments in your life. There are many ways of dealing with stress, including meditation, singing, dancing, among others. Such options will help you deal with stress and reduce the pressure on your brain. By acting to reduce pressure on your head, you respond to protect the brain and the vagus nerve as a whole.

In one research conducted by medical students from Ohio State University, it was revealed that when individual animals are put under excess pressure, they react by producing high levels of cortisol. The high degree of cortisol provided tries to reduce the volume of the hippocampus. The fact that a person is under pressure only means that they reduce their chances of having a sober brain. If you are struggling with stress, the chances are that you may not be able to concentrate or keep memories. It is essential to ensure that you reduce your levels of stress so that you focus on other aspects of life. If you do not pay much attention to your health and try to minimize the stress associated with your life situations, the chances are that you may end up living a life that painful.

All the factors that affect your brain are also impactful to your vagus nerve. Stress does not only change your mind, but it also affects your nervous system. The vagus nerve may completely fail if you keep on undergoing episodes of stress on a daily basis. The inflammation of the vagus nerve may further lead to other health complications. Swelling means that the nerve is not functioning to the maximum. A simple problem, such as inflammation, may lead to digestive and hearing problems. If the case advances, the entire vagus nerve may be affected and hence affect the autonomic nervous system.

Blood Pressure and Heart Rate

Another factor that may lead to the inflammation of the vagus nerve is blood pressure. The human body is designed to maintain a certain level of blood flow. This means that there must be signal transmission from the heart to the brain that coordinates the blood flow. The flow of the blood depends on the heart rate and the constriction of blood vessels. If blood vessels are constricted, the heart will be forced to pump the blood a lot faster so as to achieve equal distribution of blood to all body parts. In the same way, if the blood vessels are lost, the heart rate has to reduce to some extent. The vagus nerve is at the center of all the operations that affect the functioning of the heart.

Vagus nerve stimulation devices have been used for various medical purposes for more than 30 years. These devices are either implanted or used externally. Some of the joint implants are devices that range in 1 to 3.5 mA. These devices are mainly designed to influence heart rate and blood pressure. Some of the diseases that these devices aim to control include epilepsy and heart diseases. With that said, it is evident that stimulation of the vagus nerve has a significant effect on the blood pressure and heart rate.

Research shows that most of the devices used in vagus nerve stimulation, either use mechanical pressure application or automated electromagnetic waves. In the early 1800s, the data collected from such devices was vital in evaluating the overall health of the vagus nerve. Data such as the Electrocardiogram (ECG), heart rate (HR), and blood pressure (BP) were all evaluated. However, modern-day medical applications focus tends to be on the performance of the device rather than the wellbeing of the nerve. Over the years, most device manufacturers have opted to design invasive devices that do not give out data as it was initially. This does not mean that the devices used for vagus nerve stimulation are defective in any way. The main concern would be a case where the device was causing overstimulation, resulting in fatigue and injuries to the nerve.

It is recommended to use the non-invasive vagus nerve gadgets. Wearable such as the hand and thump pressure tools are much safer. Today, some manufacturers are reverting to the traditional options of belt and hand pressure. In either case, you must ensure that the gadget you chose to use has been approved and received a clean bill of health. Understanding that any stimulating device is only supposed to help you enhance activities that are already taking place will also help you understand that overstimulation may mess up with the natural processes. The human body is made to run naturally and provide internal solutions to internal problems. This explains why the vagus nerve has to defend itself from injuries. In the case of an injury, the nerve must initiate a process of self-recovery. In this process of recovery, the damages caused to the body or to the nerves must be resolved.

If you choose to use a device that regulates your blood pressure, you must ensure that it does not go beyond the required. Overstimulation of the vagus nerve will obviously lead to excessive production of some enzymes. The parasympathetic activities of the nerve are awakened during a moment when the body should be acting in the opposite direction. Although the ultimate result of reducing heart rate may be achieved, it is still expensive and painful to experience some complications associated with the stimulation. If you want to stimulate your vagus nerve for the sake of reducing blood pressure and heart rate, only do it selectively. It should not be something you do daily.

Chapter 5
Vagus Nerve and Inflammation

Let's talk about inflammation. Inflammation is something that happens in the body when there is a response to something that shouldn't exist.

Is all Inflammation Bad?

Not necessarily. Inflammation is significant for making sure you respond to different stimuli within the body correctly. With inflammation, you have either an injury, or a pain, or even an infection, and from this, you get more white blood cells, immune cells, and cytokines that are used for disease.

Inflammation is something that should be short-term, with redness, heat, swelling, and pain. But, in some cases, you might have inflammation happening within the body; without symptoms, you usually don't notice.

When there is something in the body the brain recognizes as an invader, it starts the inflammation in the body. However, when not properly turned off, it can cause a lot of problems.

What conditions does it Cause?

Well, anything that yields an inflammatory response is a culprit here. For example, diabetes, heart disease, cancer, fatty liver disease, asthma, Chron's disease, IBS, and pretty much anything with inflammation as the cause is a part of this.

Food allergies and sensitivities are also seen here. Insulin resistance is another symptom of inflammation, hence why type 1 diabetes is often a result of inflammation in the body.

While some of the inflammation can be turned off quite quickly, you'll realize that, with every single stimulus, it can actually make a lot of issues for people, and it can have a lot of problems that are very hard to fix if you're not careful.

People who are obese, or under a lot of stress, usually there is chronic inflammation there.

While you might notice it, most of the time, you have to see a doctor get some blood tests, including the C-reactive protein test, TMF alpha, and the IL-6, all of which are different chemicals that are within the body whenever you have an inflammatory response.

So, What Causes It?
Well, there are many different causes here, and the vagus nerve is actually a part of this. When the vagus nerve is stimulated correctly, it sends out the neurotransmitters to tell the inflammatory response that it's over, the invader is gone, you don't need to activate, which causes a reduced reaction.

But, with a vagus nerve that's improperly stimulated, it can cause you to have overstimulation of the inflammatory response within the body, resulting in insulin resistance, heart disease, obesity, and also other conditions.

This is partially caused by your diet, of course. Eating high amounts of sugars, carbs, high fructose corn syrup, and consuming a diet that's riddled with junk food is a part of the reason why you might have inflammatory responses, and the solution, in that case, is, of course, a diet change.

If you're stressed, and continuously activating the parasympathetic nervous system, your vagus nerve will be affected too. This, in turn, causes an inflammatory response in the body also, and hence, diseases will come forth too.

But, it's more than just the sugars. It's also how your vagus nerve is stimulated. When your vagus nerve isn't working, it won't control the inflammatory response, and oftentimes won't control the signals to the brain. This will, in turn, lead to debilitating conditions in the boy as we've tackled before.

In many instances, when we're continually reducing our "flight or fight" responses, the biological markers will help with reducing inflammation.

When you see a doctor for inflammation, chances are they won't prescribe medications for that. That's because the way to combat inflammation can't always be handled with medication, and oftentimes, drugs cause more side effects than help to the body.

The vagus nerve affects your heart rate, and also acetylcholine, which is a tranquilizer that you can administer to yourself through merely inhaling and exhaling, and from there, your parasympathetic nervous system will be activated.

When you activate this, you're essentially encouraging the "rest and digest" or the "tend and befriend" actions in the body. The "tend and befriend" actions within your organization, of course, are those neurotransmitters that are activated.

When you activate your vagus nerve, you're basically turning off all of those responses you don't need in the body, and it'll help with inflammation

Chapter 6
Vagus Nerve and Depression

When people think of mental health issues, the two that come to mind are typically anxiety and depression. Depression is the other most common mental health issue around the world, and many people suffer from it. It is estimated that somewhere around 15% of people will experience depression, either acute or chronic, at some point in their lives.

This disorder can be debilitating. It can be exhausting. It can be draining, and it can be destructive. It can lead to so many different problems, and that can be a primary reason you would benefit from trying to solve the problem altogether. Instead of continuing to stress about the issue, you can defeat the problem.

Defining Depression

Depression itself is the feeling of negativity and hopelessness that people sometimes feel. It is a period in which there is a lack of interest in the world around you. You can feel like you do not want to engage with other people. You find that anything you used to be interested in is no longer compelling. You do not want to do anything at all oftentimes, and that can sometimes really just make the problem worse.

Depression can be debilitating for these people. Especially when severe, people who suffer from depression can find they do not have the energy for anything at all. They feel slow, sleepy, even if they cannot sleep. They feel stuck and unhappy. Even the activities that once brought them joy in life are no longer enjoyable, and they find that they cannot do anything about it. This is a significant problem for people; it can really hold them back.

Depression is most often characterized by the following symptoms:

- You cannot regulate your mood up and regularly. Your attitude is frequently or always down, and you cannot figure out how to bring it back up, no matter how hard you may try.
- Your appetite has fluctuated dramatically, and you either eat more often now, or you do not want to eat at all.
- You struggle to sleep, or you sleep regularly. Either way, you always feel exhausted.
- Your mood is usually low, and you can find that you become very irritable sometimes.
- You are permanently fatigued; you cannot get yourself to move around because your body is just that exhausted that frequently.
- You struggle to really focus on what matters to you. You cannot concentrate on the most critical aspects of your life, and you feel like your mood is endlessly dull and foggy.
- You do not have an interest in anything at all, even when they used to bring you joy.
- You feel worthless, or like you do nothing but bring the world down.
- You may fixate on the idea of death or suicide.

Depression and the Vagus Nerve

Remember, when the body feels that something is entirely futile, it shuts itself off; it stops trying to continue moving forward. It finds there is no reason to stay, so it begins to shut down and slow down. When you go into a frozen state, this is what happens. Your body dulls your mind, and your concentration struggles. You lose interest and responsiveness. You feel like you cannot move at all, or like moving or doing anything at all would take far too much effort out of your life.

The vagus nerve, when it is overactive, can trigger what is known as a parasympathetic shutdown. This is the freeze response. It is a primitive response to fear, developed long before mammals developed their more modern, nuanced fight or flight system. It is believed that depression, at or at least, certain kinds of depression, may be linked to this.

There are many types of depression that can be found to be resistant to just about all treatment options—these people are known to have treatment-resistant depression, and yet, stimulating the vagus nerve has been shown to help these people begin to get back to their old routine.

It may also be the case that depression is related to inflammation, especially if swelling is treated when you stimulate the vagus nerve. Nevertheless, regardless of whether depression caused by the vagus nerve in the same way that anxiety was, one thing is known for sure—depression can be managed with the stimulation of the vagus nerve.

We are going to consider three methods that you can use to begin fighting off depression. We are going to look at probiotics—these are relevant to the vagus nerve thanks to the prominent role that the vagus nerve plays in the digestive system and the digestive system's leading role in the production of serotonin—which happens to be one of the ways that we can treat depression. We will take a look at socialization to help bring the vagus nerve back to a sense of normalcy, and finally, we will take a look at meditation.

Probiotics to Stimulate the Vagus Nerve

Every digestive system is jam-packed with bacteria. It lines most of your digestive tract, allowing your body to mainly digesting the food within your guts. The good bacteria you want to have in your intestines are known as probiotics. These are found already in many naturally fermented foods or other foods that are cultured. Take a look at the yogurt label by the time you are at the store—you may see that it is labeled as having live culture. That live culture is all of the bacteria that you can eat and then seed into your digestive system.

When you do this, you can permanently boost the power of your digestive system. Even better, however, is the fact the digestive system can realty influence your mind. Having the right gut biome is absolutely essential when it comes to being able to function accordingly. If you want to be able to perform, you must have the right kinds of bacteria to create the right types of hormones your body will need.

In particular, Lactobacillus Rhamnosus and Bifidobacterium Longum are both associated with being able to help with stress hormones. They aid in the uptake of serotonin, and they also create positive changes to the GABA, a vital neurotransmitter for general regulation. When you do not have enough GABA in your body, it may impact your mood.

While science is still attempting to determine the exact details, it is believed when you do not have enough GABA, and you could end up suffering from anxiety, mood disorders (including depression), epilepsy, and chronic pain. For this reason, it is incredibly essential for you to recognize that the gut bacteria absolutely do impact the mind, and you need to ensure you honor that.

By taking probiotics with both Lactobacillus Rhamnosus and Bifidobacterium Longum, you can ensure that your body is going to have more of those proper bacteria that it will need to not only regulate the mood but also help with the vagus nerve as well. There have been studies done that have shown that mice actually tend to show fewer symptoms of anxiety and depression when they are given these necessary probiotics, and it is believed this is due to the vagus nerve.

Socialization to Stimulate the Vagus Nerve

Once again, we come right back to the social nervous system, the proposed method through which the vagus nerve regulates the way in which we socialize. It has been found that socialization is one of the most significant ways to reduce stress, and this makes sense. Think about it—we are social creatures. If you want to alleviate stress, you need to be around people you love and care about. This socialization can leave you feeling fulfilled and better than ever.

In particular, many therapies also entertain the idea that to treat depression, you must be willing to go out on a limb and force the point. Many of them say the only way to get moving again with your own anxiety or depression is to make sure you go out. You have to sort of reboot the mind into seeing it as enjoyable and beneficial—sound familiar?

When you suffer from depression, you oftentimes do not want to do anything at all, and yet, going out there and actively beginning to stimulate your vagus nerve through being out and exposed to other people is one of the most effective manners that you can use. You need to be able to recognize the ways you can spend that time with people and how getting out there can slowly but surely begin to engage your vagus nerve.

This does not mean you have to go out to a party tonight; instead, take it slowly. Allow yourself, too, little by little, is to better cope with the way that you are behaving. Over time, you will find you are better able to focus. Over time, you will find that this time you spend out and about is worth it. You will feel like, at the end of the day, you can, and you will be able to do everything you need to do.

Get up and get out, get moving, and be social. Even if you just spend a few minutes with someone every day, having a conversation with them at the coffee shop as you wait for your order, you are still engaging with other people, and as they join with you, you will find that, little by little, you will be able to get back to functioning. You will be able to get back to feeling whole within your own body again.

Meditation to Stimulate the Vagus Nerve

Finally, the last method we are going to consider in terms of what you can do with yourself to stimulate the vagus nerve for depression is to take a look at the ways in which you can meditate. Meditation is an incredibly powerful state of mind, and it has been found to activate those same areas within the brain that are triggered by the vagus nerve as well, implying that the two are related.

When you meditate, you are entering a quiet, stable state in which you are able to relax and focus on the way in which you are feeling. You focus on the clarity and the peace within yourself, and in doing so, you are able to slowly but surely seek solace within yourself.

Meditation is something people sometimes resist, but the truth of the matter is it is actually surprisingly robust. You do not have to go out and suddenly let go of anything you enjoy to get out there and meditate. On the contrary, you can usually do it anywhere for any amount of time, with very little commitment required. All you will need is yourself and a quiet place to rest, uninterrupted, and left alone to enjoy the peace and quiet within yourself.

- Begin by finding a beautiful, quiet place for yourself where you can relax without intervention. Make sure that it is somewhere you will be able to better focus without any distractions.
- Take a deep breath in and hold it. Then, breathe out. Repeat this process, getting used to the way your breath feels.

- Find a position that you are comfortable sitting within. It could be any position at all; it does not have to be any particular one. All that matters is you are comfortable in it.
- Slowly shift your focus to your breathing. Let yourself continue to focus on just your breath at this point, paying attention to the air coming in and out of your lungs.
- Any time that you feel your attention leave your breathing, you must quietly and gently shift it back, free from any judgment and free from any concern.
- Remain in this state for as long as you feel comfortable, preferably at least five minutes.

Chapter 7
Signs Your Vagus Nerve Requires Attention

No one wants to have a vagus nerve that does not function properly. If it is as important as has been pushed throughout this, and is, you do not want to run the risk of having a vagus nerve that is not functioning well. Whether due to damage somewhere in the system or low vagal tone, you may find that you are suffering in many different ways that can be directly linked back to your vagus nerve.

The good news here is that you can treat these issues. For the most part, if you have a malfunctioning vagus nerve, you can begin to manage them. You can ensure that you are taking care of yourself to try to treat yourself better. You will be able to tap into the vagus nerve, strengthen it, and activate it to defeat this problem altogether. You will be able to ensure that you do cure yourself, and in doing so, you will be better able to cope. You do not need to get a device implanted to deal with these issues—all you have to do is ensure that you can, and do, work with yourself to treat the problem.

Vagal Tone
Vagal tone is how functional your vagus nerve is. It is incredibly essential for you to have a properly functioning vagus nerve. Still, the easiest way to tell if it is not is through tracking your vagal tone. Vagal tone is done through a test in which you can measure your heart rate variability. This is the rate at which your heart rate varies between inhaling and exhaling. When you inhale, you create a lower pressure within the chest to draw in the air. The body usually responds with the vagus nerve speeding up the heart rate. As you exhale, then, the heart rate drops as the pressure changes again. The slower heart rate means that the blood pressure can fall back to

where it should be. This is repeated with every breath you take—you see your heart rate pick up as you breathe in, and as you breathe out again, you see it dropping down back. This is seen over and over again, and the higher the difference between inhaling and exhaling, the better your vagal tone is.

High Blood Pressure

When your vagus nerve does not function properly, you will see blood pressure go up. This is due to the heart rate, not regulating itself out as much—the vagus nerve is not keeping you in a relaxed state. Because of that, you are likely to run into issues such as seeing that spike in blood pressure. When you can see that peak, however, you can begin to treat and manage it. When underactive, the vagus nerve can lead to a higher instance of the sympathetic nervous system being active. This sympathetic nervous system is what then leads to you suffering from the higher blood pressure to begin with.

Higher Resting Heart Rate

Similarly, when the vagus nerve is not functioning the way that it should be, the heart's resting rate increases. This is because the heart has its rhythm that it follows—it usually beats at a higher rate if the vagus nerve is not there to sort of regulate it and stop it from expending so much energy. This is where you get your resting heart rate—it is the heart rate at which you are calm and relaxing, and the vagus nerve is in parasympathetic mode. When your vagus nerve is inactive or weak, it is no longer regulating the heart rate at a steady resting rate. This leads to your resting heart rate ending up much higher than it otherwise would be.

Depression

Another common symptom of a problem with the vagus nerve is suffering from depression. When you suffer from depression, you are mostly stuck within an increased parasympathetic response that has then caused you to be caught in a constant, mild state of shutting down. Think of it this way—when you are depressed, and you are withdrawn. You do not want to interact with other people, and you may even feel like even getting out of bed is too much effort for you for the day. This is not because of you and your problems or because you are weak-willed—instead, it is because your brain is working against you. Your parasympathetic nervous system assumes that there is a threat somewhere and responds accordingly. The vagus nerve fundamentally fails to help you stop that parasympathetic shut down, and you get caught in a persistent state of wanting to withdraw and conserve energy. Interestingly enough, patients who have persistent, treatment-resistant depression have reported feeling better when getting vagal nerve stimulation therapy. They say a decrease in depressive symptoms that then allows them to begin exploring energized once more.

Anxiety

Another common problem that people suffer from when their vagus nerve is not functioning correctly is anxiety. This makes sense when you consider that anxiety itself is the deep, sustained feeling of being in danger. When you are anxious, it is like you hear something around you, but you cannot figure out where it is coming from. You know that there is a threat around there somewhere, but you are unsure where that threat is in the first place. That is terrifying for those suffering from anxiety—they feel like they can never relax.

Inflammation

As we have tackled, inflammation runs rampant if the vagus nerve is unable to activate for any reason, or if the vagus nerve simply does not enable. When this happens, you run the risk of inflammation running on overdrive because the vagus nerve never steps in to stop it. The vagus nerve is the part of the nervous system that will directly influence this sort of ending to the inflammation. You must be able to activate the vagus nerve to release the neurotransmitters that will alleviate the inflammation in the first place.

It is important to note that inflammation can take several different forms. Your inflammation could manifest as swollen joints or swollen parts of your body, such as arthritis. This is perhaps one of the most natural ways of inflammation to identify. However, many autoimmune disorders also carry this sense of inflammation, such as lupus or multiple sclerosis. The inflammation for these is usually a bit more downplayed and hard to identify. Still, it is there if you know what to look for.

Gastroparesis

Gastroparesis is the term to describe when the stomach becomes paralyzed in a sense. When you suffer from gastroparesis, you cannot control the movement of food from your stomach to your intestines. As a result, the food in your stomach frequently lingers without ever being pushed throughout the system. This is a scary symptom to suffer from—it can leave you struggling to digest food. When you do not digest your food, it can potentially ferment within your stomach. You also run the risk of the food solidifying in your stomach as well, and that can be dangerous.

People suffering from gastroparesis usually do so because their vagus nerve is not functioning for some reason. It could have been damaged, severing that connection that the brain used to tell the stomach to keep pushing food. The result is a stomach that will only intermittently drain or not drain at all. That is a problem—when you suffer from gastroparesis, you are at an increased risk of suffering from all sorts of issues. Such as struggling to regulate your blood sugar when the food that you eat is sporadically pushed through your system becoming malnourished or even dehydrated due to a failure to have the digestive system functioning correctly. People suffering from gastroparesis are also usually quite uncomfortable with the disorder, and it can lead to gas, bloating, feelings of fullness, and pain.

Vasovagal Syncope

Vasovagal syncope is a fancy way to say that someone has fainted. This is most commonly due to a shift in the body's blood pressure that causes there to not be enough blood at the brain to remain conscious. As a result, individual faints. This is often attributed to the vagus nerve, especially if it is in response to something scary or disturbing.

Generally speaking, the vagus nerve is meant to be a sort of regulator during periods of stress. If it sees something particularly distressing, it may overreact—it ends up trying too hard to calm down the body. Instead of only balancing out the sympathetic nervous system, it goes overboard. The heart rate then plummets, which leads to a plummeting of the blood pressure, which leads to insufficient oxygen to the brain.

This is essentially an overactive vagus nerve, and that can be a problem for you as well. The vagus nerve and its activation are situations in which you want a perfect balance of activity. Only with that ideal synchronization between the systems is that you live a healthy life.

Keep in mind that if you only occasionally suffer from this syncope, there is probably no problem. However, if you are repeatedly suffering from these sorts of events in which you randomly faint for little or no real reason, you may want to consider speaking to a doctor to ensure that there are no other causes for what you are suffering from. It is always better to be safe than sorry. You can do this in particular if you are suffering from any symptoms that may be problematic in some way for you.

Heart Takes Longer to Recover After Exercising

When your vagus nerve is not particularly strong, you will see it start to take you longer to calm down when you exercise. For most healthy people, the heart rate usually drops quite quickly after exercise—as soon as you no longer need that extended push of blood throughout the body, your heart rate begins to slow alongside with your blood pressure dropping. It will get closer to its resting heart rate quickly because it can recover from stress, both physically and mentally.

However, when your vagus nerve is damaged, it can take you far longer to calm down. Your vagus nerve may end up a bit slow on the uptake and can cause you all sorts of problems with regulation just because of that. If it cannot recognize that it is time to slow down and then activate that slowing down in the first place, it is struggling somewhere along the way and probably needs some extra help to treat it.

Insomnia

Finally, those who struggle with their vagus nerve tend to find themselves suffering from insomnia. They may find that they are actively struggling due to their anxiety being on overdrive. When they cannot activate that parasympathetic response that they need to relax and calm down to heal themselves and rest, they are going to find themselves stuck in a state of being awake. They will not be able to trigger within themselves that need to stop stressing and to relax for themselves—they will find that they simply cannot sleep, no matter how long they spend in bed.

It will only be in being able to activate the vagus nerve and tone it up to reenter that state of parasympathetic regulation that they will be able to get that critical, necessary sleep again, and that can only come with practice and treatment.

Chapter 8
Activating the Vagus Nerve and Exercises

The methods presented in this topic have been practiced since ancient times. However, given that they have zero side effects and bring about an improvement in the quality of your life, you have nothing to lose when it comes to following them.

Furthermore, it would be remiss of me not to present these exercises since all of them are talked about quite a lot. So in the interest of giving you a well-rounded look at how you can stimulate the vagus nerve, let's dive into these ancient practices.

Breathing Techniques
Humming

A dull hum can get your vagus nerve up and running. The trick is to go all out with your hum and to let your inhibitions go. It isn't so much the depth of your hum or the pitch but the degree with which you can let go. Make it as deep or as shallow as you want. The theory behind this is that the vibrations in your throat and chest will stimulate the vagus nerve since it passes through these areas of your body.

So why should you let go entirely and hum? Well, this is just to get you to give it everything you've got. Besides, everyone is different, and your vagus nerve's tuning will be different from that of others. This is why there is no standard or scale in terms of the vibrational frequency you need to hit in order to stimulate the central system.

Conscious Breathing

In the depths of my depression, if someone asked me to observe my breath, I would have thrown something at them. However, the simple act of keeping your breath has the effect of slowing it down. There are some claims that the vagus nerve is activated when your breathing slows down to seven breaths per minute.

There's no doubt that simple observation can help calm you down and will help you become more grounded in the present. There are considerable benefits to this.

Valsalva Technique

This technique is carried out by pushing your breath against a closed airway. Inhale once profoundly and close your mouth and pinch your nostrils together. Now exhale as best as you can and as forcefully as possible. This increases the pressure inside your chest and airways, and this stimulates the vagus nerve.

Given that your vagus nerve densely innervates these areas of your body, this technique is an excellent way to stimulate it.

Yoga Chanting and Yoga Poses

Activate the Diving Reflex

The diving reflex refers to the way our body reacts when plunged into the water. Blood flow increases to our brain and our senses become sharper. You don't need to jump into the water to recreate this. Simply splash your face with cold water all the way up to your eye line, and you'll feel the effects of this.

Another way of recreating this effect is to hold a pack of ice cubes against your face and hold your breath for a second. A third method is to drink water and play around with it as it flows over your tongue as you feel its texture.

Yoga

Yoga is an ancient exercise practice that originates from ancient India. It is a physical and spiritual practice that places great emphasis on learning the mind to body connection. If you really wish to get into yoga, I highly recommend locating a qualified teacher who can walk you through the various poses as well as the breathing techniques to follow.

Speaking of breathing techniques, let's look at the first practice you can follow to activate the vagus nerve.

Half Smiling

Smiling is a valuable social tool, and your ventral system plays an essential role in enhancing it. The connection works the other way as well, just as it does with socialization. Forcing yourself to smile is a great way to signal to your brain that there is no threat in the immediate environment, and it removes you from the dorsal or sympathetic nervous state.

This isn't a yoga practice, and you can do this wherever you are, as you go about your day. Move your mouth into a half-smile, and imagine your jaws loosening. You can close your eyes if you want when doing this.

Opening the Heart

Sit down on the floor and close your eyes. Bring your hands to your shoulders and inhale deeply. As you inhale, open your chest and raise your head and simultaneously rotate your shoulders outwards. As you exhale, turn your shoulders back in and lower your chin into your chest.

Perform this movement a few times and make it as smooth as possible. This relaxes the muscles in your neck and lower head and, as a result, relaxes the nervous system as well.

Warrior Pose
=====

The warrior pose isn't a terribly complicated pose, but it is best if you learn the posture from a teacher who can explain the intricacies of it to you. The pose brings your breath and body into sync and forces you to ground yourself to the earth. It also tests your ability to balance and is a great way to start off your day.

Cow Pose
=====

You can perform the cow pose by kneeling down on a mat and then supporting yourself on all fours as you extend your hands out in front of you. Tuck your stomach in as you inhale and bend your neck inwards. As you exhale, let go of your belly and arch your back and shoulders down as you look upwards.

The vagus nerve innervates your belly, and as a result, this pose helps activate it.

Metta Meditation (Loving-Kindness Meditation)
Metta refers to loving-kindness, and this form of meditation has been shown to place the mind in a state of mind that promotes peace and love. The meditation itself is straight forward. Close your eyes and take a few deep breaths to ground yourself in the present moment. Once this is done, visualize all the people in your life and send them all the love you have and wish them well.

Then, visualize someone you don't know and have never met and send them the gift of your love. Visualize yourself, showering them with all your love and compassion. Practice this for five minutes and observe the difference in your mental state. From a biological perspective, loving-kindness meditation helps remove yourself from a country where a threat exists to an environment where you are safe and secure. This naturally helps activate the ventral system.

Yoga Nidra

Nidra is usually the culmination of all yoga practice sessions. To do this, you simply lay down on your mat or on the floor with your palms facing upwards. Observe your breath and the sensations in your body. Practice this for around 10 minutes or so.

Other Factors That Stimulate the Vagus Nerve

The following factors aren't confined to yoga or any particular exercise method but nonetheless have an effect in stimulating the vagus nerve. Where applicable, I'll highlight research that supports the benefits of these methods. You can and should implement all of them immediately

Singing

I've already asked you to hum, so you might as well sing at this point. It doesn't matter how atrocious you are, and singing helps you activate the vagus nerve. Just like humming, the key is to truly let yourself go and sing at the top of your voice. Medically speaking, this stimulates the muscles at the back of your throat and helps activate the vagus nerve better.

Meditation

Like yoga, meditation is a practice that originates in ancient India. Meditation's benefits extend well beyond stimulating the vagus nerve. Meditation has been shown to literally change your brain and rewire it to create a greater sense of calm. As far as anxiety and depression are concerned, the increased awareness that meditation brings can be a problem since it will make the problem appear worse at first.

The key is to have a strategy in place beforehand that you can carry out. Remaining detached and observing or reinforcing positive habits at this juncture are examples of things you can do to implement change.

Laughter

Laughter is extremely beneficial for your well-being, but you don't need me to tell you that. A study conducted on people practicing yoga laughter (an exercise where you throw your hands up and laugh as hard as you can) found that their Heart-Rate Variability decreased. As you've already learned, HRV has a direct correlation to vagal tone. The lower the HRV, the higher the vagal mood, and the better health you are in.

Prayer

A study conducted on those performing rosary prayers found that their vagal tones increased. The exact reason for this is not known. There is speculation that counting the beads produces changes in the breath and that this is the cause of increased vagal tone.

Pulsed Electromagnetic Field Therapy

This method involves sending electromagnetic waves through the body with an aim to stimulate bodily function. A study conducted on healthy, middle-aged men found that PEMF therapy resulted in increased vagal tone. You can buy devices off the shelf that provide such stimulation.

Probiotics

As mentioned, the gut microbiome plays an essential role in regulating your mood and the consequent anxiety and depression levels. Probiotics help with this, but keep in mind that most supplements are of no use. It's far better to consume fermented foods such as yogurt or sauerkraut to help with digestion.

Exercise

Perhaps the best medicine of them all for anxiety and depression. Exercise and physical movement challenges you and gives you a sense of accomplishment, which directly opposes the miserable feeling that depression causes. In case of anxiety is your issue, exercise gives you an opportunity to vent your frustration at something.

Exercise also releases endorphins in your system and helps you feel better. All in all, there is no downside to exercise, and you should aim to make it a part of your daily routine.

Massage

A massage is a form of visceral manipulation, and a full body massage relaxes you entirely and removes any blocks in your body. Certain types of massages directly stimulate the vagus nerve and are incredibly beneficial for your health.

Fasting

Fasting helps the body regulate the production of ghrelin in your system, and this helps regulate your blood sugar as well as your metabolism. In addition to this, practices such as intermittent fasting help you lose fat and increase muscle tone, which enables you to become healthier.

Sleeping on Your Right

Research is pretty limited with regards to this, but there is anecdotal evidence that is sleeping on your right increases vagal tone. There's nothing to lose by trying this out to be honest.

Recommended Foods

Seafood

Seafood happens to be rich in Omega 3 fatty acids that play an essential role in diminishing free radicals within our system. Free radicals are a blanket term used to describe chemicals that cannot be flushed out by the body on its own. They've been linked to the existence of cancer and other autoimmune diseases.

Fiber

Fiber helps with excretion and improves gut health. Given the gut to brain connection, consuming fiber in your diet should be a priority.

Sensory Deprivation

Sensory deprivation is a method that has been increasing in popularity lately. The technique is best suited for people who do not have claustrophobia, and there is significant research that suggests that the technique works exceptionally well.

To begin with, the method itself is pretty straightforward. It works by immersing yourself in a highly concentrated salt and magnesium bath. This allows you to float in the water entirely without any aid and thus creates a sense of weightlessness. Your eyes will be covered, and you will shut the lid of the tank on top of you. Keep in mind there are also open-air tanks that don't have caps for those of us who like a little bit more breathing room.

Chapter 9
Passive Method to Activate the Vagus Nerve

Besides all the active exercises you can perform on your own, there are passive treatments that can have profound effects on vagus nerve activation. Some of these involve using specific equipment or visiting a health care provider. In contrast, others can be done in your home comfort. Before beginning any treatment, remember to discuss these options with your primary health care provider.

Auricular Acupuncture

A substantial and increasing body of research indicates that in many patients with depression, anxiety, epilepsy, LPS-induced inflammation, tinnitus, and highly active pain receptors, acupuncture and transcutaneous vagus nerve stimulation through the auricular branch of the VN produce positive results. The best part about this form of treatment is that it is efficient without invasive action.

Visceral Manipulation

Visceral manipulation (VM) is a less common therapy, but it is highly effective when correctly practiced. Typically practiced by osteopaths, chiropractors, naturopaths, and other health care providers, VM is the gentle physical manipulation of the abdomen's organs, increasing the flow of blood to areas that do not function best. Once learned right, patients can use this feedback device on their own.

All abdominal organs, including the liver, gallbladder, pancreas, kidneys, spleen, stomach, small intestine, and ascending and transverse parts of the large intestine, are innervated by the vagus nerve. For the VN to influence these organs and communicate organ function to the brain, the proper functionality of the organs is essential. In these organs, physical restrictions can build up, which can only be altered by material manipulation and mobilization. Improving the blood flow to these organs can have significant beneficial organ health outcomes and allow the VN to send out optimum function-related signals.

Gently administered hands-on treatment is used by visceral stimulation practitioners to find areas of change or reduced activity within the viscera to remove constraints within these visceral organs. The therapy involves gentle compression, mobilization, or soft tissue elongation. Having a licensed emotional stimulation specialist in your region may be a good idea, especially for those with detoxification disorder or liver, gallbladder, or kidney discomfort.

Electrical Stimulation
Researchers have performed experiments in the last hundred or so years to learn about the symptoms of the vagus nerve. One technique involved stimulating the VN on experimental animals with the aid of electrical stimulators. In addition to learning about the value of the VN itself, researchers eventually determined that they were able to supplement its functions by electrically stimulating the vagus nerve.

Experiments were done in the 1980s and early 1990s to show that vagus stimulation in the neck was effective in reducing seizure activity in dogs. This research resulted in dedicated clinical trials which produced devices for vagus nerve stimulation (VNS) that could be implanted into the neck. The FDA approved these devices for the treatment of epilepsy in 1997, and the treatment of chronic, treatment-resistant depression in 2005. Regarding various medical problems, including insomnia, bipolar disorder, treatment-resistant anxiety disorders, Alzheimer's disease, and obesity, laboratories and companies have been developing and enhancing tools to activate the VN since electrically. The most widely used clinically electrical VNS system is the Cyberonics NCP Program, which is inserted during an outpatient procedure on the left vagus nerve. This unit is used for treating patients with severe depression and epilepsy resistant to the treatment.

Right-side VNS is effective in animal models of epilepsy and seizures. Still, substantial effects on depressive symptoms are not known. Preliminary human trials are promising and have produced positive results, and some firms have already started to create vagus nerve stimulation tools that can be used for different conditions. BioControl Medical's CardioFit system uses right-side VNS to activate efferent fibers and help in heart failure treatment. In contrast, BioControl Medical's FitNeSS system is designed to activate afferent fibers, thereby helping to reduce the side effects of electrical vagal stimulation.

Typical surgical risks associated with this procedure include infection, pain, scarring, swallowing difficulties, and paralysis of the vocal cord. Side effects of implanted electrical stimulators include voice changes, heaviness, sore throat, cough, headache, chest pain, breathing problems (especially during exercise), difficulty swallowing, abdominal pain, nausea, skin tingling, insomnia, and bradycardia (heart rate slowing). Though many of these may be temporary, they may be severe and may last forever.

Other electrical stimulation systems do not need to be implanted. Still, they have mixed results and are only licensed at this stage for specific conditions. Cerbomed's NEMOS system is a transcutaneous VNS unit, applied to the vagus-innervated portion of the body. Currently, it has been cleared for epilepsy and depression treatment in Europe. In Europe, gammaCore device from the US-based company electro Core has been granted clearance for acute treatment of headaches in clusters, migraines, and overuse of problems by medication. The gamma Core is a portable handheld device with two flat contact surfaces for stimulation that are applied over the vagus nerve to the neck side. More extensive trials for treating other conditions are underway.

Daily Practices for Activating the Vagus Nerve

- Gargling 2x daily: Keep a cup to your sink. Use it to rinse your teeth twice a day, in the morning and at night.
- Gag reflex activation 2x daily: Use your toothbrush to activate the gag reflex on both the left and right side of your soft palate, as you brush your teeth in the morning and at night.
- Humming 2x daily: Practice humming deep in your mouth during your daily commute, or to note your day. You can use the term "om" to keep the pulse as long as you can exhale in your throat.
- Cold shower 1x daily: End your daily shower with cold water for one minute (as cold as possible) and practice breathing through the temperature change shock. It becomes easier to increase the time every three days by 30 to 60 seconds until all of your showers are taken under cold water.
- Deep breathing 3x daily: Before each meal, perform three to five minutes of deep breath in a quiet room. This will help calm you down for each meal and improve your digestion.
- Sunlight exposure 3x daily: Go outside and expose your skin to the sun within 30 minutes of sunrise, in the middle of the day, and within 30 minutes of sunset, at least five minutes each time. If you live in a colder climate, expose your eyes to the light for two to three minutes at each of these times and practice breathing through the cold whenever you do so.
- Sleep on your side each night: Put a pillow in between your knees to prevent you from sleeping at night on your side.

Chapter 10
Creating a Vagal Tone Routine

To get the best results for your vagal tone, you can create a daily routine. However, here are some points that you should remember when you are using a method. The whole point of the routine is just that; it should happen regularly. So try and incorporate those activities that you are comfortable doing. Do not try to cram too much into your day, or else you might find yourself unable to perform certain operations. This, in turn, might demotivate you. You need to feel a sense of accomplishment, so make sure you are comfortable performing the activities every day.

Start with a few simple additions to your life. This way, you will make it seem like there are no significant changes in your life. You do not disrupt anything, but at the same time, you are stimulating your vagus nerve every day. But that does not mean you should not focus on making the other activities and processes as part of your life. As you keep getting used to certain habits, think of ways you can incorporate the other practices. Remember, all of them don't necessarily have to be done every day, as we are going to see.

Each of the routines below will increase in complexity. Get used to one before you move on to the other.

With those four quick tips, let us get started on the routines.

Routine #1
This is a relatively easy routine that you can perform. When you wake up in the morning, make sure that you rinse after you have finished brushing. If you are grazing in the evening, then you can even rinse again once you are finished.

This is the simplest of the routines. You might already be rinsing after brushing. The only difference is that you should try and extend to about 20-30 seconds, rather than quickly rinsing and spitting out the water when you wash your mouth.

Routine #2
In this routine, you can start splashing your face with cold water. Now you might wonder why I didn't just combine this with the first routine. The main reason is that many people prefer to wash their face with lukewarm or warm water.
Once you are used to Routine #1, you can add splashing your face with cold water to your daily habits.

Routine #3
We are going to add breathing exercises to the mix.

As soon as you wake up in the morning, practice the Deep Breathing Technique for about 10 minutes. As I mentioned earlier, don't worry if you are unable to do it correctly. What matters is that you get started. You will eventually be able to master it.
If you have 30 minutes in the morning, you can start by practicing the deep breathing technique for 10 minutes and then move on to yoga for about 20 minutes.
At this point, your routine should look like this:
Morning

- Wake up and then Deep Breathing Technique (with yoga if you have 30 minutes)
- Rinsing after brushing your teeth
- Splashing cold water on your face

Evening

- Rinsing after brushing your teeth

Routine #4
You start by waking up in the morning and head out for a brisk walk or jog after the sun has risen.

You come back and rinse after brushing your teeth. You then splash cold water on your face.
Once you return home in the evening, you then practice the Deep Breathing Technique or yoga,
You then end the day by rinsing after brushing your teeth.
The above routine might be a bit too overwhelming for some. So if you feel that you are unable to keep the above method, then make sure that you use Routine #3 but then alternate between yoga and brisk walking.
So your new routine might look something like this:
Morning 1

- Wake up and then Deep Breathing Technique (with yoga if you have 30 minutes)
- Rinsing after brushing your teeth
- Splashing cold water on your face

Morning 2

- A brisk walk outside after the sun has risen
- Rinsing after brushing your teeth
- Splashing cold water on your face

Evening 1

- Rinsing after brushing your teeth

Let's plug that into a timetable and see how it looks.

Days	Morning Routine	Evening Routine
Monday	Morning 1	Evening 1
Tuesday	Morning 2	Evening 1
Wednesday	Morning 1	Evening 1
Thursday	Morning 2	Evening 1
Friday	Morning 1	Evening 1
Saturday	Morning 2	Evening 1
Sunday	Morning 1	Evening 1

A simple timetable will allow you to get all the benefits for your vagus nerve.

Routine #5

This is the most advanced routine. But, essentially, what we are going to do is create two morning routines and two evening routines.

We need to start adding a relaxation routine and one for laughter. When it comes to relaxation, pick up an activity that you can use to unwind. It could be reading, listening to wonderful music, or even cooking, if that relaxes you.

So essentially, you are going to have the below options to work with.

Morning 1
- Wake up and then Deep Breathing Technique (with yoga if you have 30 minutes)

- Gargling after brushing your teeth
- Splashing cold water on your face

Morning 2
- Brisk walk outside after the sun has risen
- Gargling after brushing your teeth
- Splashing cold water on your face

Evening 1
- Unwind with a relaxing activity
- Gargling after brushing your teeth

Evening 2
- Tickle your funny bone
- Gargling after brushing your teeth

Let's plug them into a timetable and see what happens.

Days	Morning Routine	Evening Routine
Monday	Morning 1	Evening 2
Tuesday	Morning 2	Evening 1
Wednesday	Morning 1	Evening 2
Thursday	Morning 2	Evening 1
Friday	Morning 1	Evening 2
Saturday	Morning 2	Evening 1
Sunday	Morning 1	Evening 2

Remember, you can sometimes combine a few things. For example, you could be someone who unwinds by watching comedy. That is a beautiful idea too. However, some people enjoy reading a book more than watching something funny. To them, having a separate day for getting a laugh is essential. If you can combine relaxing and laughing, then that would also be doubly beneficial. However, I am going to assume that you are busy with a lot of other vital chores or responsibilities.

One of the best things about the above routines is that you can change and modify them to fit your purpose. So you could add a gentle Deep Breathing Technique in the afternoon along with Routine #2 if that is possible for you. I would recommend that you do not think of the routines as rules established in stone. They are more like notes you make on Google Docs; you can change them easily.

Make sure that you try and incorporate all the methods that improve your vagus nerve. Too busy to do yoga every day? Try every weekend. Not a morning person? Then the morning Deep Breathing Technique is perfect for you!

Chapter 11
Meditative Techniques for the Support of the Vagus Nerve

We've already tackled some of the great benefits of mindfulness meditation. It can help you focus on your present moment and make you more aware of your body. It can bring awareness to physical sensations you would have ignored before. All of this can help you further understand your physical reactions to stress and how to bring relaxation to your body. There are many different ways you can approach meditation. Choose the one that you're the most comfortable with.

One mindfulness meditation that can help with stress, anxiety, and depression is loving-kindness mindfulness. This is because it creates more positive emotions, which, in turn, change your body physiology and help you improve your vagal tone. Loving-kindness can help you overcome any issues with low mood or low self-esteem. They can also help you with emotions like anger, guilt, and resentment. All of these involve our feelings about ourselves or others. Loving-kindness is about reminding yourself of kindness to you and others. It creates so many positive emotions that it can change your mentality and is a great way to start improving your cognitive distortions.

To start your loving-kindness meditation, you're going to need a safe, comfortable space. Since this meditation is kind of long, you may want to have this book open while you do it, or you can listen to a guided meditation to walk you through it. This loving-kindness meditation is based on the work of Dr. Emma Seppala.

Start by sitting cross-legged if you can or sitting on a chair. Relax your body, and close your eyes so that you are focused on your inner world, rather than the external one.

1. Take a deep breath in and slowly release it.
2. Think about someone who is close to you and loves you. This can be someone from your life now, someone from the past, or someone who has passed away. Imagine that person standing beside you.
3. They are sending you their love and their hopes for your happiness and safety. See and feel the warm wishes coming from that person toward you. You might picture it as a wave coming toward you, filling you, and surrounding you.
4. Think about a second person who also loves you. They also send you their love and their hopes for your happiness and safety. See and feel that warmth surrounds you and enter inside of you.
5. Now, imagine that you are surrounded by all the people you have ever known who love and cherish you. Your friends, family members, and community are sending you their love and their hopes for your happiness and safety. Surround yourself in that love and fill your heart and body with it. You are overfilled with love.
6. Look at the first person beside you. Start to send them your love. You and this person are alike; you both wish for happiness and love. Send your love and your hopes for their pleasure and safety to them.
7. Silently repeat this phrase three times, sending the wishes to that person.
    - May you be safe, may you be happy, and may you be healthy.

8. Now focus on the second person on your other side. Start to send them your love. You and this person are alike; you both wish for happiness and love. Send your love and your hopes for their pleasure and safety to them.
9. Silently repeat this phrase three times, sending the wishes to that person.
    - Like I hope to, may you live a good life full of safety, happiness, and good health.
10. Now imagine all of the other people who love you. Start to send them your love. You are all alike; you all wish for happiness and love. Send your love and your hopes for their happiness to them.
11. Silently repeat this phrase three times, sending wishes to those people.
    - May your life be full of happiness, well-being, and health.
12. Think of an acquaintance that you know. Someone that you have no particular feelings toward. You are all alike; you both wish for happiness and well-being. Send all of your hopes for their well-being to them.
13. Silently repeat this phrase three times, sending the wishes to that person.
    - Just like I hope to, may you live a good life with health and happiness.
14. Think of another acquaintance who you know, but don't have any particular feelings toward. You are all alike; you both wish for happiness and well-being. Send all of your hopes for their well-being to them.
15. Silently repeat this phrase three times, sending the wishes to that person.

- May your life be full of happiness and well-being.
16. Now imagine the whole world in front of you. All of the living beings in the world are just like you; they all want to be happy. Send all of your warm wishes to them.
17. Silently repeat this phrase three times, sending your wishes to every living being in the world.
    - May your life be full of happiness and well-being.
18. Gently bring your awareness back to yourself. Take a deep breath in and then out. Bring awareness to your body and mind. Think about how you feel after doing this meditation. Open your eyes and continue your day.

Once you've completed the meditation, you should feel a little better. You may feel relaxed and calm. You may even feel more compassion for others. If you don't, that's okay. Keep practicing loving-kindness meditation to gain the benefits from it. If this isn't your cup of tea, try some other kinds of meditation. If you want a more physical sort of meditation, try yoga, qigong, or taiji (Thai chi).

Yoga is often considered relaxing as it uses movements and breathing to help calm the body. It can sometimes be triggering for people, so if you've experienced trauma or PTSD, proceed with caution or do yoga with someone who understands trauma. There is some evidence that yoga can stimulate the parasympathetic nervous system and the Vagus nerve. It's also been linked with helping to heal depression, anxiety, stress, and chronic pain. So it can be worth it to try if you want to activate your Vagus nerve.

There are a lot of different types of yoga to try. If you've been practicing yoga for a while, stick with the ones you know or try something new. If you're a beginner, then don't start with the advanced classes.

Here are some significant types of yoga that are good for beginners but also help with stress reduction:

Hatha Yoga - In a hatha yoga class, you'll have a basic understanding of the different poses in yoga. It's generally considered to be a gentle yoga class and shouldn't strain you too much. You'll learn to work on posture, while also following the breath.

Iyengar Yoga - This type of yoga is very focused on your position and poses. There isn't a lot of strenuous work, but you'll have to maintain poses for a while. The classes should be run by someone who understands the human body well and can provide you with support in different positions. If you choose to do Iyengar yoga, make sure that your instructor has been well-trained and can provide you with the necessary guidance, so you don't hurt yourself.

Restorative Yoga - Like the name itself suggests restorative yoga is all about relaxation. In this style of yoga, you put yourself in poses while being supported by other materials. So while you are in the pose, you're not straining yourself.

Each of these kinds of yoga can require a class with an instructor. However, if you don't want to go to an actual level, you can find some good yoga videos online. For relaxation, choose yoga videos that use terms like gentle yoga, beginner's yoga, or yoga for relaxation. Find videos that you enjoy and help you relax. If gentle yoga is not your thing, they try vinyasa yoga, ashtanga yoga, or Bikram yoga. All of these are more intense, but also put a lot of emphasis on the breath and movement. All of them can help you achieve more balance in your body.

Qigong is a new type of meditation. It combines physical form and movement with focused breathing and meditation. Its goal is to balance your life energy or Qi. It has a lot of backing from both traditional medicine and modern science. Many scientists consider qigong to promote well-being. It causes relaxation of your muscles, reduces your stress levels, and deepens your breathing, which has been repeated many times thus far and can help with activating your Vagus nerve. Qigong has many different forms, and it can be adapted for many different people. It's often used medically in China, is related to many kinds of martial arts, and is sometimes just simple meditation and movement. One of the most popular forms of qigong in the U.S. is tai chi.

If you've ever walked through a park in a major city during the weekday morning, you may come across a group of people doing slow, fluid movements that look very much like martial arts. They're most likely doing Thai chi. It is, in fact, a type of martial arts that focuses on the body's slow movement and breath. It is considered a style of meditation, even though there is an exercise component to it. If you're interested in either qigong or tai chi, find a class near you and give it a try. You can also find videos on YouTube for home practice.

Tai chi takes a lot of practice before its flow becomes routine, so keep working with it.

Chapter 12
Measuring Nervous Function with Heart Rate Variability (HRV)

Vagal tone refers to the effect that is created by the parasympathetic nervous system on the body at rest. It affects the heart rate, lungs, and digestive tract.

Put merely, and vagal tone is how the parasympathetic nervous system responds to stimuli. The reaction that we humans give when stressed, sick, or traumatized is affected by the parasympathetic and sympathetic parts of the autonomic nervous system. The parasympathetic system influences are, however, more prevalent. Vagal tone is often used to determine heart functionality and emotional regularities.

Vagus Nerve Testing
To check whether your vagus nerve is underperforming, a health practitioner might test your gag reflex. They do this by irritating the back of your throat. If you do not gag, it could be down to your vagus nerve not working in the manner in which it should.

Measuring your vagal tone is a bit more complicated than tickling the back of a person's throat. Testing your vagus nerve's strength includes monitoring your heart rate variability (HVR).

HRV looks at how fast the body boots into the parasympathetic nervous system response of "rest and digest." The higher your HRV is, the higher your vagal tone will be. It suggests that having a high vagal sound causes a person to experience far better moods, health, and brain function.

An electrocardiogram can measure your heart rate. Did you know that when we breathe in, our hearts beat faster to speed up oxygenated blood throughout our bodies? When we breathe out, our heart rate automatically slows down again. The vagus nerve is activated when we breathe out but impaired when we breathe in. These differences in heart rate indicate your vagal tone. In plain English, it means that your body can deal with stress and is capable of processing stressful situations faster.

If you experience a low HRV, you will have a low vagal tone. Those who have low HRV or vagal tone take far longer to recover from illness, stress, and situations that cause unease and discomfort. Low HRV is sadly also linked to inflammatory diseases, cancers, heart diseases, and brain conditions. That is why there is a considerable impact that stimulating the vagus nerve can have on overall health and treating illnesses.

A Closer Look at Heart Rate Variability (HRV)
These days, we can track all sorts of bodily information, such as sugar levels, weight, and the number of steps we did. By monitoring HRV, a person may soon be able to discover the impacts that stress has on the body and its effect on energy output and more. HRV is there to monitor the fluctuations in time between each heartbeat. The variations, as mentioned in the discussion about vagal tone, are controlled by our autonomic nervous system, so even if we want to react in a certain way, our bodies usually respond in a manner that is out of our control.

In saying so, the autonomic nervous system is forever working, and messages are being relayed back and forth between the brain and the organs to gauge and weigh our experiences and then provide the body the opportunity to react in what it thinks is the appropriate manner. If we experience continual stress, live a rather sedentary life with no exercise, and do not sleep well, combined with dysfunctional relationships and lousy eating, the body will try to balance itself out, causing our flight-or-fight reactions more prevalent. Think about how happy you are when you get a raise or when your first child is born. All these feel-good moments will impact your health in a more positive light and cause the right reactions.

Why Should I Check My HRV?

Checking your HVR is a great way to test the autonomic responses within your body. If you find yourself more in a flight-or-fight mode, naturally, the fluctuations between heartbeats will be lower. Relaxation brings with it higher variations between heartbeats. Low HRV levels bring a myriad of problems, including cardiovascular issues, and it can exacerbate depression.

If you have a high HRV, you will be able to handle stressful situations with a lot more ease and experience better cardiovascular fitness. By monitoring your HRV, you can make small improvements that can significantly benefit you throughout your day and lifetime. Through simple practices such as meditation and practicing mindfulness, HRV rapidly improves. There is definitive proof that this is something that people should learn more about and invest. HRV can be the reason you change your life for the better!

HRV Testing

HRV can be tested in the doctor's rooms by attaching wires to a person's chest and monitoring the fluctuations. The relayed data is then printed on a sheet of paper that the doctor then reads, thus determining HRV. HRV can be tested at home, too, with a chest-strap heart monitoring system. It is advised that you check your HRV right after you wake up during the week to gauge where you can make changes to your lifestyle to improve your health.

Chapter 13
(VNS) Vagus Nerve Stimulation

Alternatively, several home-based methods can also be used to stimulate this nerve. When a device becomes needed, it is usually to treat cases of epilepsy and depression that haven't been able to respond to other medical treatments such as pharmaceuticals or psychotherapy.

The device is located under the skin of the chest or neck, with a wire connecting it to the vagus nerve itself. The device can then send signals through the vagus nerve to your brain stem and then process the information given to your mind. The device would typically be programmed and controlled by a trained neurologist. Still, the patient will often receive a handheld magnet that can also help them manage their equipment. Studies are being conducted currently with the hopes that in the future, the stimulation of the vagus nerve can also be used to treat other conditions such as Alzheimer's disease, migraines, and cluster headaches, as well as multiple sclerosis.

We all know the saying, "What happens in Vegas, stays in Vegas."

Well, things tend to work a little differently when we refer to the vagus nerve. What happens in the vagus nerve most certainly doesn't stay in the vagus nerve, no matter how much you try to keep it there. Stimulation of the vagus nerve can affect just about the entire nervous system, as it links the brain to the heart, lungs, and digestive tract.

It also goes a step further and allows interaction with the liver, kidneys, ureter, female fertility organs, neck, spleen and gallbladder, ears, and the back of your tongue. It also helps to release bile and testosterone into the system as well as stimulate the secretion of your saliva and release tears.

When the vagus nerve gets damaged or has a problem, there can be many physical issues abnormally slow heartbeat, weight gain and obesity, gastrointestinal disorders and diseases, trouble swallowing, mild to severe mood disorders, fainting spells, seizures and epilepsy, vitamin deficiencies, and chronic inflammation within the body.

By stimulating the vagus nerve, we have found that we can improve on certain conditions such as the following:

- Heart disease is a condition involving blood clots to the heart as well as diseased blood vessels and structural problems with the heart itself.
- Tinnitus causes a buzzing or ringing sound in your ears that you may associate with hearing loss. This ringing noise may be a constant sound, or it may come and go.
- Obesity is a condition of a person's weight. They fall on the larger end of the scale and develop other secondary issues on top of their weight.
- Alcohol addiction where a person ultimately becomes utterly dependent on alcohol to function in society.
- Migraines are painful headaches, often causing a loss of balance, eye sensitivity to light, as well as seeing 'spots' or patterns in vision.
- Anxiety disorders whereby a person may experience intense and uncontrollable feelings of worry, stress, or fear to the point that it interferes with the person's daily routine in society and leaves them unable to function correctly.
- Alzheimer's disease is a progressive disease that takes over a person's mental functions and destroys their memory.

The leaky gut syndrome is a gastrointestinal digestive condition where toxins and bacteria can 'leak' through the intestinal wall, affecting the rest of the body.

Inadequate blood circulation is often caused by a buildup of plaque within the arteries and blood vessels, resulting in stiffness in your limbs as well as severe pain.

Mood disorders are classified generally as extreme highs or extreme lows. This is an elevation or lowering of someone's mood for a short period.

Cancer, whereby abnormal cells within the body will uncontrollably divide themselves and destroy body tissue and healthy cells along the way.

With vagus nerve stimulation, we can say that approximately 80% of nerve fibers are meant to send information from the body and organs to the brain. In comparison, the other 20% of nerve fibers will send data back from the brain to the rest of the body.

Your daily diet can also play a significant role in how your vagus nerve functions and is stimulated.

A healthy diet is more likely to leave you feeling energized with your vagus nerve getting all the power it needs to function. In contrast, a junk food diet that consists of high-fat and high-carbohydrate meals will reduce the nerve's sensitivity overall. Eating overly spicy foods can also cause the vagus nerve to have a moment of miscommunication with the body.

So, since the vagus nerve has control over such a vast amount of our gastrointestinal tract, we can say that when a person has a 'gut feeling,' they are feeling it in their gut.

It isn't just in their imagination, as these nerve signals that we feel control a vast amount of our lives to keep us safe and healthy. These feelings come from the vagus nerve that is telling us that there is a chance that something in the current situation might be wrong.

Your gut feeling is due to a part of the nervous system being stimulated that precisely controls your gastrointestinal tract called the enteric nervous system. This nervous system then communicates with the brain via the vagus nerve.

It has also been found that up to 90% of the main signals and communication that is passing through the vagus nerve is coming from the enteric nervous system firing away.

Medical professionals have been studying the vagus nerve's influence on the human brain thoroughly, especially in the sense of using electrical stimulation to help combat the effects of epilepsy or depression. Vagus nerve stimulation is now able to help prevent a person from getting seizures by sending mild electrical pulses to the brain regularly, using a small device that is implanted under the skin.

It has also been found, especially with patients who have epilepsy, that this device has another added benefit that goes along with it, which is that these patients felt like their mood had drastically improved after using the machine, showing that the benefits of helping those who are depressed can also be achieved.

Vagus nerve stimulation can also be achieved using passive methods such as holding your breath for a short period, splashing cold water over your face, coughing suddenly, or even squeezing and tensing the stomach muscles in a bearing down motion.

Concentrating on your breathing through meditation is a gentle and passive way to stimulate your vagus nerve and become more self-aware of all that is around you. You could join a yoga class or meditation class that can explicitly teach you these specific breathing exercises.

Alongside the vagus nerve stimulation therapy, you can also get vagus nerve blocking therapy, which is similar to using the stimulation device but will only be used during the day. With vagus nerve blocking, you are blocking specific signals to the brain instead of stimulating them.

For example, you can block the signal that tells your brain that you are hungry and therefore need to eat something. Instead, the vagus nerve bypasses that particular sign. Your mind will not get the message that you are hungry, thus reducing food intake during the day. This appropriate method is often used in obesity cases, allowing the patient to curb any unnecessary cravings.

The vagus nerve has now also been stimulated to help patients who have epilepsy. This form of epilepsy treatment was first performed in 1997, through the vagus nerve stimulator device being placed into a person's chest under the skin and a wire linked to their vagus nerve. When stimulating the vagus nerve electronically for the treatment of epilepsy, the patient may find a few side effects that may become uncomfortable. Should the following side effects be experienced, the patient should visit a doctor immediately to see if there is a way to reduce or stop the symptoms.

- Hoarseness or changes in voice - The patient's voice becomes quite rough and grainy, sounding, which can ultimately lead up to our symptoms.
- Sore throat and difficulty with swallowing - The patient may experience pain in their throat that will also affect their speech and daily functioning.
- Coughing - can lead on from the sore throat. The patient may experience a 'tickle' or rough sensation as they speak, which triggers the gag and cough reflexes.

- Shortness of breath - The patient may find that since their vagus nerve stimulator is also directly linked to their diaphragm, they may experience some discomfort in breathing and not be able to get the lung capacity that they may just have had.
- Slow heart rate - As this little artificial ticker sits in the chest cavity controlling your vagus nerve, it will also monitor your most crucial ticker, the heart. The parasympathetic side of the vagus nerve will be stimulated, thus slowing your heart rate as if you had just been in fight or flight mode, it is time to relax.
- Stomach discomfort or nausea - This comes from that nasty 'gut' feeling we tackled earlier. Your digestive tract reacts to the vagus nerve being stimulated. It may make you feel quite ill as if you were going into a situation you'd rather not be a part of.

If any of these problems continue to occur during your epilepsy treatment, please inform your doctor as soon as possible.

Because the vagus nerve has connections to every organ in the body, researchers now think that the vagus nerve might be able to help other cases and reduce nasty symptoms along the way.

These studies are now being performed on heart failure patients, those with diabetes, abnormal heart rhythm, Parkinson's disease, as well as severe inflammation from Crohn's disease. When it comes to such cases as those with arthritis, which affects most of the population at some stage in their lives, studies that were done in 2016 showed that the symptoms of arthritis could be significantly reduced with the stimulation of the vagus nerve. The patients who did not respond to medications for their aches and pains showed significant improvement after vagus nerve stimulation. No adverse side effects were shown as a result of the trials.

Chapter 14
Practical Exercises to Stimulate the Vagus Nerve

The Power of Stretching

Let's talk about stretching. This doe tie into yoga, but if you combine diaphragm breathing with yoga. Doing this as you do a mall stretch will benefit you in a ton of different ways. For starters, most people don't stretch nearly enough, and it shows. Most people aren't flexible, and it affects how they end up faring in life. Many get injured due to a lack of stretching.

But it's more than that. Stretching is powerful. Stretching is used to help naturally stimulate the body, and make movement simple. There is a lot you can get from this, and you can get out of this. Most people don't realize that they're not only releasing tension within the muscles when they stretch, but they're also focusing their breathing, so it's simple and yet very useful.

A lot of people don't stretch enough, so that tension sits there. But, a way to naturally start up the parasympathetic nervous system and activate et vagus nerve is to do just this. Sitting down, stretching out your body, and working on this helps promote relaxation and wellness, and from there will stimulate your entire body in its way.

Plus, it feels fantastic too. Most people don't stretch enough, and they'll realize as they do this, that they need to. Sometimes having calming music, and focusing on your breathing changes this.

You also don't have to hold the stretches for very long. About 10-12 seconds suffices.

Try touching your toes, stretching your arms behind your head, pushing them up, and holding your arms in the air, or even just moving towards your foot will help with this. There is a lot of benefits to be had with stretching and a lot of beautiful things to do with this. You'll be shocked, you'll be amazed, and most of all, you'll be quite happy with the power of this small exercise. You'll feel invigorated for whatever is to come for you in the future.

Consider stretching right before you begin your day, or at the end of the night, and see how it helps you feel during the day. You'll feel your vagus nerve stimulate almost immediately.

Weight Training

Weight training might seem weird to do to stimulate the vagus nerve, but it does work. That's because, when you lift weights, it is changing the speed of the body. Plus, through the power of repetition, you get your body to relax. A lot of people think lifting weights is only for big, burly people, but that isn't the case.

Ever just doing a few sets of curls will change the way your body feels, and your vagus nerve. Many people also think they need to start with a heavyweight right away, but that isn't the case. I suggest just progressively overloading over time if you want to see physical gains. You must understand that weight training is a relaxing process, and you must breathe as you do it. You need to breathe in deeply to help with pushing the oxygen around to help you with strenuous exercise. So yes, pick up that dumbbell and try it. You'll feel the difference right away.

HIIT Workouts

HIIT, or "high-intensity interval training" is a form of workouts that require you to do a lot in a minimal period. Sometimes, this involves sprinting; other times, this can be pushups, sit-ups, or other exercises. The main goal behind this is to do a lot in a bit of time, and through spurts.

These sprits are what cause vagus nerve stimulation. The vagus nerve is usually not stimulated if you're always stressed out. Still, the periods of stress, and then relaxation kick the vagus nerve into gear, helping it activate whenever needed.

HIIT workouts are also great because they are often straightforward to do. No matter what it is that you do, you'll feel the difference in these immediately.

A lot of people don't realize that HIIT is also very short in terms of workouts.

Some people can get these done within a half-hour or so, and that's their workout for the day. But HIIT is great because it lets you get a great workout and also lets you improve your wellness and health.

It's a great way to get in shape, so it's something you should consider if you're looking to improve your physical fitness.

Walking

Walking is an excellent option if you're not going to the gym to lift or don't want to spend time doing HIIT or yoga. Walking is an excellent habit to get into because it stimulates your body and helps with physical fitness and wellness. Your vagus nerve will get stimulated with walking, especially if you live a sedentary lifestyle.

I think walking for 30 minutes a day is ideal, especially if you're unable to do this otherwise. Sometimes, pacing while on your breaks is a great way to do this, and walking also lets you improve on your health and wellness.

You want to do this to help with your physical fitness, and walking is a good start, especially if you're not active otherwise.

Jogging is also another good one because this can help with deep breathing. A lot of people, when they start, will get into the habit of breathing with short breaths, but that won't work here. This can make it hard to run, and you might pass out. With jogging, you want to make sure that you're breathing in a slow, deep, and even manner, and focus on this. This will help with your vagus nerve and help you get into the habit of breathing deeply. You can also do running with this, but it's more high-intensity and might be harder to engage in deep breathing otherwise.

Jumping

Again, another form of cardio that's great, but your vagus nerve will love it. Jumping jacks, burpees, and other jumping exercises are useful because they help improve circulation, which can help with blood pressure and your vagal tone.

When you jump too, be mindful of your breathing. Try to do it with a deep breath, and you'll notice it's a much harder workout, but you'll feel the difference. It increases blood flow, blood pressure, and heart rate as well.

Your vagus nerve will thank you for this, and you'll be able to, with jumping too, improve on your health and wellness.

Aerobics

Aerobics is another higher-intensity exercise, but some variants aren't as extensive or intensive as others. Zumba tends to be on the more intensive side, but there are different classes you can try. However, there are even different kinds of aerobic exercises, such as water aerobics, weight training, cycling, and even yoga.

All of these, when combined, are wonderful for vagus nerve stimulation and are great for the body. You'll be amazed and surprised at how helpful this can be for the body, and how you can use these to help improve your vagus nerve. They encourage you to breathe during these too, which promotes deep breathing and thereby vagus nerve stimulation.

Swim it Out!

Swimming is a great aerobic exercise too, and if you're not a fan of jogging or running, or weight training, swimming is good.

That's because it helps in many different ways. For starters, you're submerging your head, which stimulates the mammalian diving reflex, which includes your vagus nerve. It also pushes you to control your breathing as you move. You need to hold your breath, but also walk through the water, and it's a combination of both of those things which provides you with the correct vagus nerve stimulation.

It also will help improve your bodily movement. That's because you're moving about, and this encourages blood flow too. You'll notice that as you begin with this, it's hard to do, but over time, you'll get better with this. It's a beautiful form of cardio, and it's gorgeous for properly stimulating the vagus nerve.

Dancing

Finally, we have dancing. Dancing is an excellent form of self-expression for starters. Even if you're silly, it can help you feel much better about yourself. Dance is lovely because it enables you to improve your physical fitness, get the blood flow moving, and help you stay active and fun.

There are so many different kinds of dance classes these days too. You can do Zumba or other forms of dancing. Some people even like ballet dancing because it requires control, and this can stimulate the vagus nerve. They're fun to do, and they encourage you to move, control your breathing, and let you express yourself.

Even silly interpretive dancing helps. After all, if it can make you laugh, that naturally stimulates the vagus nerve, and that's a beautiful, fun way to do this.

Dancing is excellent, and it lets you feel good about yourself. Consider dancing the other time you want to express yourself correctly and feel good.

When it comes to stimulating the vagus nerve, these are all practice activities that boost the vagus nerve. Your vagus nerve is vital because it lets you relax the body and helps curb inflammation. But, while these exercises are great for stimulating this, it also helps with getting the body moving, which increases vagal tone. It can also help offset obesity, diabetes, and other conditions related to weight.

Your vagus nerve does benefit from exercise, and here, we tackled why and how it happens, and the benefits of this.

Chapter 15
Health And Life Benefits of Vagus Nerve Stimulation

Vagus Nerve and Depression

Depression, or major depressive disorder, is a mood disorder that causes a person to have persistent feelings of sadness and loss of interest. Depression can affect a person mentally and physically and take a significant toll on a person's daily activities. It is an illness, just like any other, that can cause a person just not to want to face life and become secluded. Even though mental health is gaining prominence and becoming accepted by the general population, a significant segment of the population does not take it seriously. They feel that a person can just snap out of it. This is not the case. A person cannot just snap out of it. Depression is more than just getting over something. It is an illness that may require medical attention. There is a difference between having an off day, and a major depressive disorder that significantly reduces your ability to function every day. When a person is suffering from severe depression, they are often walking a thin line, and one little thing could push them over the edge. For this reason, their feelings and mood disorders always need to be validated. They need to be taken seriously.

Untreated depression can lead to significant pain and trauma. Severe depression may lead to a person harming. There are many unfortunate stories of people who did not reach out for help, out of fear of appearing weak, and things took a turn for the worse. We do not want this to happen to anybody because they felt like they could not reach out to someone. Depression is not something to take lightly, and if a person is exhibiting the signs of depression, it must be taken seriously. There are many signs and symptoms of depression that must be considered. Among them are feelings of sadness and tearfulness, anxiety, reduced appetite, unexplained physical problems, feelings of worthlessness, seclusion, loss of interest, anger, frustration, always blaming themselves, and many other things. Take special notice when someone suddenly stops doing something they have always loved to do. Also, give special attention to significant mood swings.

A study conducted in 2002 in biological psychiatry showcased outcomes that long term vagus nerve stimulation vastly improved symptoms of major depressive disorder and reduced episodes of depression. Stimulation of the vagus nerve appears to change brain wave patterns, which reduces the symptoms of depression. This implies a significant physical component for depression. However, doctors are still not fully aware of exactly how vagus nerve stimulation improves symptoms of depression. It just seems to work well, which is a good thing. Perhaps there is a connection between an overstimulated sympathetic nervous system that speeds up body processes and depression. This is something that is still not fully understood. One thing that researchers want to emphasize is that stimulating the vagus nerve may not eliminate depression. However, it will always vastly improve a person's quality of life. If a person can at least feel good most of the time, then a particular therapy is worth paying attention to.

Other times a person you know and love is experiencing symptoms of depression; don't get annoyed. Depression is an illness, just like diabetes, and a person suffering from it needs support, and not be told to just get over it. Perhaps using the natural techniques for vagus nerve stimulation may be beneficial for them. Once again, it may not cure their depression, but it will improve their mood and ability to live life tremendously. If vagus nerve stimulation continues to inhibit depression effectively, then maybe the stigma that still exists around mental illness can be eliminated once and for all. This just may be the most significant result of all. Even people who have mental illness feel guilty. We don't hear people apologizing for heart disease. But they still apologize for being depressed. This needs to stop, and increased vagus nerve research can help.

Here is one suggestion that will help all parties involved. When promoting a friend who is experiencing depression, take them out to have some fun. Remember that laughing and having a good time helps to stimulate the vagus nerve. Take your friend out for a night on the town, and you may just help with their depression.

Vagus Nerve and PTSD

Post-Traumatic Stress Disorder, or PTSD, is a mental condition caused by a traumatic event that had a severe impact on someone. The people who are affected most commonly are in the military, law enforcement, first responders, or anyone in a field where tragedy is a common occurrence. However, PTSD may also strike just about anybody and everybody who has been through a traumatic event. A serious accident, death of a loved one, getting assaulted, or any number of tragic events may cause a person to have PTSD. It may take years to overcome PTSD, and some never overcome it at all. PTSD can manifest itself in multiple ways, including anxiety, anger, nervousness, negative thoughts, flashbacks, and chronic pain. They will often re-experience the trauma various times in their heads. There is a significant split, even within the military community, whether or not PTSD is legitimate.

For this reason, just like with depression, people will dismiss it as a non-issue. They believe that someone can just get over it. A person cannot only get over it, though. PTSD is genuine and is a severe mental disorder that needs to be treated as such. Unfortunately, PTSD continues to carry a negative stigma to it that can hopefully be a thing of the past once people start realizing some of the physical elements to it as well.

While there is no known cure for PTSD, there are therapies that may be used to help subside some of the signs and symptoms. Currently, some of the treatments include talk therapy and exposure therapy. Several studies suggest that vagus nerve stimulation may be a productive adjunct therapy for helping with PTSD, especially with its associated pain. A University of Texas, Dallas, and study researched the effects of vagus nerve stimulation on rats. The rats in this particular study were shown to display some signs that come with PTSD, like fear, aggression, and anxiety. A session of vagus nerve stimulation showed a significant reduction in these negative signs. Not only that, but the symptoms also did not return in many cases after another episode of trauma, suggesting that the stimulation may have more long-term effects than the other therapies. Researchers feel that if the stimulus can work in the same manner in humans, it may significantly reduce the pain associated with PTSD. If the effects are more long term as well, it is undoubtedly an adjunct therapy worth looking into.

If you have a friend or loved one who experiences PTSD, perhaps it is time to work on them. Help them by using the techniques that will stimulate their vagus nerve. That old cliché of "laughter is the best medicine" may be the ultimate tool. Help your loved one get regular exercise. Remember, this does not just mean going to the gym. Most people are more likely to do something if they enjoy it. Find something they want to do physically and help them do it. If they love playing basketball, play a quick pickup game. If they love going for walks, find a beautiful trail, and enjoy the sites. Whatever you can do to get them moving, do it. Finally, how about a nice round of karaoke? Singing and dancing are a great way to stimulate the vagus nerve and get your friends out of the poor mental state. If we can continue to correlate vagus nerve stimulation with helping to subside the signs of PTSD, we can hopefully remove the stigma associated with it. Just like with depression, we may never be able to cure PTSD, but we can certainly manage it with the appropriate practices.

We want to talk about how PTSD can manifest itself into physical symptoms like muscle tightness, chest pain, fatigue, and digestive issues. Many of these physical responses to a traumatic event indicate a sympathetic nervous system activity. Things like muscle tightness and chest pain that is not heart-related often come from stress and being worked up for so long. They do not come from being in a relaxed state. Furthermore, fatigue develops when the body is overly stressed for long periods. This is why excessive sympathetic responses are not healthy for the organization. If your body is in a constant state of pain and tiredness due to a traumatic event, then perhaps it is time to stimulate your vagus nerve to inactivate your parasympathetic response. The parasympathetic response inhibition will put your body in a state of relaxation, releasing the built-up tension and helping reduce the pain associated with PTSD. Do this regularly, and it can help to manage the negative signs and symptoms of Post-Traumatic Stress Disorder.

Vagus Nerve and Inflammation

Does the vagus nerve help with inflammation? Yes, it does. Inflammation, also known as the inflammatory response, is your body's natural response to a variety of things, such as stress. The inflammatory response occurs under many circumstances, especially when our body is trying to fight off disease. Mild inflammation is needed for the body to maintain its proper functions. When the body perceives a threat like an illness or injury, the inflammatory response kicks in to subdue the threat. This can be marked by swelling, pain, fevers, and fatigue. Once again, inflammation is needed to help out bodies maintain their functionality. However, excessive or untreated inflammation can create many health problems throughout the body. In cases of stress, inflammation may occur due to the sympathetic nervous system's fight or flight response. In general, whenever the body perceives any type of threat, it inhibits the parasympathetic nervous system. It stimulates the sympathetic reaction so that it can deal with the perceived threat. This is why you will notice an increase in heart rate when a person has an infection. The body is becoming stimulated to defend itself.

Vagus Nerve and Stress

Stress is a significant trigger for the inflammatory response also. Indicating even further, the sympathetic nervous system is at play here. In this case, things like deep breathing and humming will effectively reduce stress, inhibit the sympathetic response, stimulate the vagus nerve, and ultimately reduce inflammation. When encouraged to its full potential, the vagus nerve can strongly influence the immune system, thereby affecting good health. The vagus nerve is looking more durable and more energetic, the more we talk about it.

One of the words we have continuously used is the word "help." We have said that the vagus nerve "helps" the human body. We say this because the vagus nerve alone cannot just solve all of our problems. At least, not at this moment. Stimulating and utilizing the power of the vagus nerve is more of an adjunct therapy for improving body processes and preventing chronic diseases, both physically and mentally. We don't want it to sound like a cure-all. Of course, it will cure a lot. Allow your vagus nerve to "help" you feel better. The point is to make the vagus nerve work as efficiently for us as possible.

Chapter 16
Vagus Nerve Stimulation to Heal from PTSD

Stimulating the vagus to stop the sympathetic system is done when the individuals feel safe and secure. The following activities can instantly promote varying levels of these feelings.

Make connections with others. It is challenging to feel as if you can trust others. The best way to switch from the sympathetic nervous system to the parasympathetic nervous system is to make a connection with someone else.

Hug. Along with the first technique, hugging helps us feel safe and connected to others. By giving or receiving a hug, you can instantly trigger the vagus nerve.

Laugh. If hugging is not your thing, you can laugh instead. Laughing can help stimulate the vagus nerve to release oxytocin. Oxytocin encourages you to make connections with others and lift your mood. Laughing, just like hugging, helps you feel connected with others and can strengthen bonds.

Shake it off. One of the ways you can bounce out of the shutdown mode is to do a full-body shake. Before you go into a full out shake, do a quick body scan. Are there any areas of your body that feel tense or stiff? If you find tension in your body, these are the areas you want to focus on when you wiggle and shake. Give your attention to each area as you shake the tension out when you have gone through all the fields and feel relieved, pause for a moment to take in the stillness that surrounds you and let it fill you. This is your body waking up again. This is the feeling you want to recall when facing a trauma-induced memory or episode.

Daily Long-Term Vagal Toning Technique for Trauma and PTSD

Healing from trauma or PTSD can be a life-long process. Strengthening the vagus nerve daily results in developing the skills necessary for your mind and body to bounce back from traumatic events and experiences that trigger trauma symptoms. The following regular exercises you can perform to receive long-term benefits from the vagus nerve:

1. Bhramari pranayama. The Bhramari pranayama is referred to as the humming bee breath in yoga practice. This type of breathwork helps you tone the vagus nerve by stimulating it through the vocal cords. When you perform this breath, you can keep the nervous system calm and prevent it from going into fight or flight mode. To achieve this type of breathwork, get into a comfortable sitting position on the floor or bed. Cross your legs and bring your hands to cover your ears. Your thumbs should face down towards the ground. Take a deep breath in; as you exhale, begin to make a humming sound that vibrates through your ears. You can repeat this process as many times as you need.
2. Sleep on your right side. Trauma and PTSD have severe adverse effects on sleep, and how you sleep can add to these difficulties. Sleeping on the right side of your body can stimulate the vagus nerve and lead to a more restful night's sleep. You should avoid sleeping on your back as this is often the worst position for vagus nerve stimulation.

3. Tai chi or qigong. Like yoga, tai chi and qigong are forms of slow movement exercises that stimulate and tone the vagus nerve. These practices focus on strengthening the internal systems through precise moment and breath. Sun Style tai chi is a type of tai chi that utilizes smooth, flowing movements that can help individuals feel grounded. This is an essential aspect for those with PTSD who can often feel lost and unsure of where they are, resulting in panic, frustration, and confusion. Doing a simple Sun Style tai chi sequence can tone the vagus nerve and be an effective way to help heal from trauma.

Sample Short Form Sun Style Sequence:

Step 1: Begin at a standing position with the elbows near your side, slightly bent upwards. Palms should face in towards each other. On the exhale, lower your arms and your bend your knees slightly, then lift the arms back up as you take a step forward on the left foot. Push your hands in front of you as you bring the right foot up to meet with the left. Feet should be slightly apart.

Step 2: Bring the hands back slightly towards the chest, palms facing one another. As you inhale, move them wider apart; on the exhale, push the palms back in towards each other.

Step 3: Step the right heel slightly up and out to your right side. Allow your weight to shift to the right leg as you turn your palms to face out in front of you. Push the palms forward, then extend the arms around and out to your side. Your gaze should follow the left hand. Then bring the palms back around in front of you, so they face each other again while stepping the left foot up to meet the right. Bend the arms, so they are at a 90-degree angle in front of you. Fingers should point toward the ceiling.

Step 4: Move the right hand to meet the left elbow. Step your right foot out to your right side as you move your right hand to extend in front of you, palms facing away from your body, and the left arm comes down. Shift your weight from your right leg to the left leg as you turn the upper body slightly to the left and move the right arm down somewhat to your side while lifting the right wing with the palm facing away from your body. Bring the left foot closer to the right and repeat this process two times.

Step 5: Bring the hands back slightly towards the chest, palms facing one another. As you inhale, move them wider apart; on the exhale, push the sides back in towards each other.

Step 6: Shift your gaze to the right hand as you stretch it out in front of you while the left hand comes to meet the right elbow. Step your left foot out to your side as you reach the right hand up towards the ceiling. Turn the left palm to face the floor and push down towards the ground. Your weight should be on the left foot. Turn your body slightly to your left as you move the left hand to sweep across your left knee and bring the right hand towards the right ear's side. Push the palm of your right hand forward and deliver the right foot in just barely to meet the left.

Step 7: Bring the hands towards the center of the chest, so the palms are facing each other (about 6-inches apart). Move the right hand forward as you step back on the right foot. Keeping the weight on the right foot, bring your left foot back to meet the right as you move the right hand back and bring the left hand forward.

Step 8: Step forward on the left foot while turning the palm of the right hand up toward the ceiling and the left palm down toward the ground.

Shift your weight to the right foot as you move your right palm out in front of you and the left palm back toward your abdomen. Bring the right foot forward, stepping in front of the left while reversing the palms so the remaining faces towards the ground and the right up towards the ceiling. Shift your weight to the right foot as you move the right hand back towards the abdomen, and you left out in front of you. Step the left foot in front of the right as you make your hands into fists and bring the right-hand level with the left.

Step 9: Bring the left foot back slightly. Un-fist your hands and turn the palms, so they are facing out in front of you. Step back on the right foot as you push the hands forward. Shift your weight to the right foot and bring the sides back in towards your body.

Step 10: Turn the palms, so they face one another. On the inhale, move them wider apart; on the exhale, push the hands back in towards each other.

Step 11: Repeat all the above steps but start on the reverse side.

Chapter 17
Vagus Nerve Stimulation to Heal from Trauma

The body experiences other distressing signs of post-traumatic stress— a tightness in the abdomen, a sinking sensation in the stomach, a familiar pain in the mouth, or a constant sense of fatigue. We now understand that as part of the recovery process we have to turn to the body and as a result, we have seen an increase in the use of meditation, mindfulness, tai chi, qigong, Feld ink circle, massage, Craniosacral therapy, dietary therapy, and acupuncture for post-traumatic stress disorder.

Such mind-body treatments are helping us to be less passive, less aggressive, and less impulsive to stress. We're growing our understanding of the options we need to make us stay grounded and relaxed. We felt in need of this more. One way the mental-body treatments operate is by activating the nerve in the vagus. Awareness of how this nerve works offers a profound understanding of traumatic stress and promotes our healing capacity. The vagus nerve has, therefore, taken center stage in the treatment of trauma.

"Mind-body treatments work on the nerve of the vagus to help you regain the balance—some breath and movement activities in this article, aimed at relaxing and resetting the vagus nerve. By a cycle of self-study and conscious body consciousness, you will continue to develop techniques that help you regain a sense of comfort and recover from trauma." Effects of Mind-Body Therapy Vagus Nerve Yoga Dr. Arielle Schwartz. The utilization of mental-body therapy is correlated with a wide variety of wellness and wellbeing changes, including physical and mental wellbeing enhancements Reduction. They allow us to focus on our feelings, impulses, and behavioral motives. This observational capacity tends to improve tolerance to discomfort, which can reduce emotional reactivity, fear, panic, chronic pain, and depression. Mind-body treatments improve self-understanding and the capacity to perceive that person's point of view with understanding.

Moreover, mental-body treatments are successful as they require structural improvements in the autonomic nervous system as determined by increases in vagus nerve activity. The vagus nerve reaches through the muscles of the nose, inner ear, chest, back, lungs, stomach, and intestines from the brainstem down. Mind-body treatments make changes in how we relate to our surroundings by encouraging a gentle look and allowing us to try new breath or activity patterns that communicate specifically with other parts of the body. Researchers also calculate the changes that exist in the vagus nerve, which is often referred to as respiratory sinus arrhythmia by heart rate variability (HRV). HRV refers to the rhythmic heart rate oscillations that arise with the breath. It's a function of the intervals between beats in the heart. Higher variability in heart rate is associated with a better ability to withstand or rebound from stress.

In comparison, lower variability in heart rate is correlated with stress and anxiety. You should think of any form of mind-body therapy that improves the heart rate variation by creating strength and endurance within the autonomic nervous system. As a result, switching between emotions of anticipation and easiness is smoother.

Pain and recuperation of the vagus nerve vagus and pain. If we feel a threat (real or perceived), we change the way we breathe. We can get a good picture here by considering the ways animals react to predators. In certain situations, an animal may rapidly breathe into the upper chest, which is a protective reaction of the nervous system that allows them to run or fight in a dangerous environment. In other situations, an object may freeze that includes breathing shallowly or holding the air to prevent a predator from being detected. This freeze reflex causes the animal to stand very still and is a response to the threat of immobilization. For certain situations, animals are weak, and a predator, not a scavenger, can lose interest in a dead animal. An evolutionarily older vagus nerve axis supports both the freezing and sluggish responses as a member of the parasympathetic nervous system.

Most notably, an animal can activate the stress reflex by shaking and breathing in a manner that maintains homeostasis until it's healthy. Nevertheless, we humans will also live for long periods either in high activation (fight and flight) or weak activation (freeze and faint) responses. This appears to be the case where abuse is persistent and prolonged, as in the case of Complex PTSD (more of this can be found here). We frequently miss the resources to handle challenging or painful experiences. It may result in physical stress and restricted breathing habits that form the foundation of our posture, modes of activity, and general self-sense.

The Vagus Nerve and Trauma Therapy

To help repair the vagus nerve, you will learn practices; but, not all training is right for everybody. Alternatively, I encourage you to play with and try a range of methods of breathing and action before you discover what fits for you. You will start developing techniques through a cycle of self-study and conscious body consciousness that help you maintain a sense of protection and recover from trauma. Here are a few tools to help get you started: Attend your Gut: Dr. Arielle Schwartz Somatic Therapy. You can also boost the health of the vagus nerve by ensuring a balanced digestive system. The inner nervous system, also known as the belly brain, is comprised of the "microbiome" that resides in the gut. This habitat includes hundreds of healthy and bacterial organisms that live within the intestinal tracts. An imbalance in your intestine can result in an inflammatory reaction in your immune system and cause a wide range of debilitating symptoms, including anxiety and depression. By raising the sugar intake and finding any latent food intolerances, you will build a balanced microbiota. You may require a doctor or nutritionist to help find the causes of a deficiency in the gut; however, the effort it takes to incorporate these improvements into your life is well worth it.

Conclusion

Chronic pain and inflammation is a terrible condition to live with. Still, as everything has shown, there is hope in the incredible power that the vagus nerve holds. The truth is that vagal stimulation is still in its infancy. Research is continually being carried out and the areas of potential research. As mentioned, merely scratch the surface of the full body of new studies that are being undertaken. You can expect this decade to bring rapid advances in the field of chronic inflammation remedies, and the vagus nerve is likely to be at the front and center of it. Living with pain is severe. It's even worse when you realize that all those pills you're popping aren't doing anything for you and are mere placebos. It is a position in which my wife and I found ourselves at different points in our lives. Thanks to the miracle that is the vagus nerve, we managed to dig our way out of it. Challenges in life never cease, but living with pain, inflammation, and chronic illness is one particular challenge you don't have to deal with day in and day out. While the vagus nerve is a miraculous thing, it helps to live a healthy lifestyle. As you can see from the alternative methods to stimulate the vagus nerve, the majority of solutions point towards living a balanced and overall healthy lifestyle. This is precisely what ancient wisdom teaches us, and we would do well to follow it. Methods such as yoga and meditation might not find an excellent fit for themselves in today's reaction based medicinal approaches. Still, when it comes to being proactive with regards to your health, they remain amongst the best solutions to undertake.

So take action starting right now and begin implementing the stimulation exercises mentioned. I can guarantee that they will change your life for the better. After all, everything is the result of meticulous scientific research I carried out to heal my family's conditions. In other words, healing the vagus nerve means treating the body. Your entire being is so intimately connected that it almost seems silly to look at your body as a series of separate parts. Stop thinking of yourself as a machine that needs to be fixed and is thinking of yourself as a living being, the product of thousands of years of evolution. Your body is perfectly adapted, in some sophisticated ways, to survive and thrive here on planet earth. It has far more healing power than you may have ever given it credit for. While its design may not be perfect for handling social media interactions or supporting you forty hours a week in your office chair, it's designed is perfect when supported by a whole and healthy lifestyle. Please don't blame yourself or your body for its physical, psychological, or emotional shortcomings. Instead, work together with your body to gain autonomy over your wellness. Protect and nurture your body, unleash its rejuvenating power, and begin to see your body as a partner in the healing processes, rather than the cause of all your troubles. It will take time for you to reap the benefits but never lose hope that better days are ahead. One of the benefits of vagal stimulation is that as your mood improves, you'll begin to believe in the treatment to a greater extent. This will create a self-reinforcing positive cycle.

I wish you the best of luck in your path forward and look forward to hearing your story of how you banished pain, inflammation, and chronic illness away from your life. Good luck and I wish you all the health in the world!

Printed in Great Britain
by Amazon